FEAR PROOF

FEAR PROOF

THE COURAGE TO LET GO, BEGIN AGAIN AND DO IT SCARED.

JAXON FEELEY

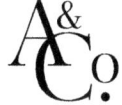

First published in Great Britain in 2025
by Authors & Co.
www.authorsandco.pub

Copyright © Jaxon Feeley 2025

Jaxon Feeley asserts the moral right to be identified as the author of this work in accordance with the Copyright, Designs and Patents Act 1988.

ISBN 978-1-917623-19-3 (paperback)

All rights reserved. No part of this book may be reproduced or transmitted in any form or by any means, electronic or mechanical, including photocopying, recording, or by any information storage and retrieval system without the written permission of the author, except where permitted by law or for the use of brief quotations in a book review.

To my family - my everything, my roots, my rocks, my why.

To my friends - for holding me up and standing by me through every scary moment.

To my dogs - for saving my life more times than I can count.

To little Jess - who never gave up, and thank God she didn't.

CONTENTS

Introduction ix

PART ONE
THE UNRAVELLING

1. Trapped 1
2. The Grace to Grieve 17
3. Things to Keep, Things to Lose 31
4. The Quiet 44
5. The Climb 62

PART TWO
THE BECOMING

6. Choosing to Leap 77
7. The Fear Spectrum 84
8. Living By Design, Not Default 93
9. Beyond the Quiet 99
10. The Climb Back Up 115

About the Author 121

Fear Proof 'fɪə / 'pru:f *(adjective)*

1. The state of mind where fear is no longer the barrier, but the compass.
2. The ability to feel fear fully, without letting it dictate your choices.
3. The practice of meeting risk, uncertainty, and emotional exposure - and moving forward anyway.
4. A way of living built not on the absence of fear, but on the courage to act alongside it.

Fear Proofing 'fɪə / 'pru:fɪŋ *(verb)*

- The process of letting go, beginning again, and doing it scared.

INTRODUCTION

DO IT SCARED – WHY I'M HERE WITH YOU

When I was about six or seven, I was a bridesmaid at my auntie's wedding. I cried all morning. Not because I didn't love my auntie, I did. But because she was making me wear a dress. I didn't want to wear a dress. I wanted to wear my football kit.

My mum battled with me to get me dressed, and afterwards she knelt to my level and said, "Sorry, darling. Just for one day, you need to wear this dress."

So I did what any determined little human would do: I wore the dress.

And hidden underneath it? My football shorts.

That night at the reception, my mum lifted my dress to fix the under gown, and there they were, clear as day, my shorts. Every adult around me burst out laughing because that was just who Jess was. Fiercely determined to do what felt right and true to me, even if it didn't fit the occasion.

That kid? She's still here. She just grew up, changed her name to Jax, and took on some bigger challenges than sneaking football shorts into a wedding.

I've been through more reinventions than I can count, some by choice, some because life gave me no other option. I've battled crippling anxiety, questioned who I was and where I belonged, served my country, faced some of life's most dangerous people and places, rebuilt my life from scratch, and was forced to make decisions that scared me to my core. That's the short version.

And here's what I've learned: the good stuff is *always* on the other side of the thing you're scared to do.

That's why I wrote this book. Not because I think you should live like me, but because I know how it feels to live a life that doesn't fit, and how terrifying and liberating it is to start building one that does.

You don't have to be fearless to change your life. You just have to do it scared. Do it scared, over and over again.

The right decision often feels uncomfortable, uncertain and risky, but that's usually the decision that will change your life.

This isn't a book of motivational fluff. You won't find airy metaphors – mine are very functional – or 'just think positive' advice. You'll find practical tools, real stories, and honest conversations about what it takes to stop living on autopilot and start living on purpose.

You already know the thing you need to do.

It is the thing you keep postponing. The conversation you're avoiding. The change you've been secretly dreaming about.

Stop waiting to be 'ready' and take that first step, football shorts and all. That's what this book is to help you do.

But Why Listen to Me?

I've lived through the stuff most people hope they never have to face and have come out stronger on the other side. I'm not a celebrity. I'm not a billionaire. I'm not here because life's always been easy.

I've touched down in Iraq with a rifle in my hands and walked the streets of Sierra Leone during the Ebola crisis. I've been threatened with blades and pool balls in socks, and I've pulled back prisoners from the brink of an overdose. I've transitioned in the public eye, spoken on stages and shared my story with millions of people. I've faced the kind of fear that makes your hands shake and your voice break, and I've learned how to move forward anyway.

This book is about you, not me. But if my story and the lessons I've learned can help you see your own courage more clearly, then every hard thing I've done has been worth it. I don't have all the answers, but I know how to find them when it matters. I know what it's like to stand at a crossroads between the life you're living and the life you want and to take the path that scares you.

So let's get to work.

PART ONE

THE UNRAVELLING

Every life-changing story begins the same way, with something breaking.

Sometimes it's loud: the shattering of a relationship, the collapse of a career, or a single moment when the fragile life you've been holding together with both hands finally slips through your fingers. Sometimes it's quiet: a whisper in the back of your mind you've been drowning out for years, until one day, you can't.

'The Unravelling' is that part. It's the breaking point, the messy, raw, terrifying beginning. No one posts about this part because there's no neat bow on it yet. There's just you, standing in the wreckage of what you thought you had to be.

In these pages, you'll see what happens when the armour comes off. When the performance ends. When you're left with nothing but the truth you've been running from and the smallest flicker of something you didn't expect to find here…

Hope.

I won't lie to you – this part is hard. It will test every reason you have for changing your life. But if you stay with me through the unravelling, you'll see why it's the most powerful chapter of any transformation.

Because when everything false falls away, what's left is real.

And that's when the light comes back into your eyes.

1

TRAPPED

WHEN FEAR BECOMES A CALLING

The Edge

If you've ever smiled for the world while quietly breaking inside, this chapter is for you.

There comes a moment. It's not always loud or dramatic. Sometimes it's just a quiet tightening in the chest, a sensation you can't quite name but can't shake either. You realise you can't stay where you are, but you also have no idea where else to go. And yet, if you're willing to keep walking with me, I'll show you exactly how to get through this. More than that, I'll show you not only how to survive it, but how to come out the other side as a person unrecognisable to the version of you who's reading these words right now.

It's like standing barefoot at the very edge of the top of a cliff in the middle of a storm. The wind doesn't just blow, it bites. It whips up the kind of cold that gets into your bones and makes your teeth ache. The salt in the air floods your mouth and nose. The sea below, hidden beneath a blanket of low cloud, crashes against the rocks in a relentless, urgent rhythm that thuds like a warning. Your toes grip the rough, wet stone.

Behind is the life you know: familiar, structured, perhaps 'successful' by other people's standards. Instagram-worthy, perhaps. There's safety there. But deep down, something aches. You've outgrown it, or it's outgrown you. You feel the urge to leap.

Ahead of you is a vast, terrifying unknown. You can't see what's beneath the clouds. You don't know how far the fall is, or what's waiting if you jump. It is the chasm of uncertainty we all fear. You don't even know if your landing place will be better than where you are right now, teetering on this cliff. All you know is that something inside you whispers, "There's more than this." When your gut keeps whispering that there's more, it's not lying. The truth is relentless like that; it keeps knocking until you open the door.

Your leap doesn't come out of nowhere. It builds quietly through your discomfort and the resentment you're too polite to voice. At first, you tell yourself you're just tired. You call it a bad week, a bad month. Then you avoid certain people because you can't fake the smile anymore. Your playlists change. Your sleep changes. You stop making plans. But the knot in your stomach doesn't loosen; it tightens. One day, the weight of pretending is heavier than the fear of letting it all go.

Pause for a second. Think about the last time you felt that quiet pull. Not the obvious kind, the one no one else saw. The details matter. Where were you? What could you hear? Your body remembers even if your mind tries to forget. Did you feel it in your stomach, your chest, or somewhere else entirely? Keep that moment of feeling the pull in your mind as we keep going. If you've got a pen, write it down.

Maybe for you, the edge isn't a cliff at all. Maybe it's a very literal situation, sitting in your car outside work, knowing you can't face another meeting. Maybe it's lying in bed next to someone you no longer recognise. Maybe it's staring at your bank statement, realising you've built a life you can't afford, not just financially, but emotionally. Whatever your edge looks like, you'll know by the knot in your stomach and the quiet thought you can't unhear.

I think of a woman who sits in her car every morning outside the supermarket where she's worked for fourteen years. She grips the steering wheel until her knuckles turn white, talking herself into walking through the door one more time. She doesn't hate her job, but she knows it's slowly eating her alive, bite by bite, day by day.

You already know what it is, don't you? The one thing you've been avoiding, excusing or dressing up as something else?

And that whisper? That's what starts to shake your world when you thought you'd built the life you always wanted.

Standing on the edge, your heart beats louder than your thoughts and a lump you can't swallow down forms in your throat. A thousand 'what ifs' pull at your ankles, all at once. Peering over the edge brings the guilt of wanting more than the life others would be grateful for. And worst of all is the fear that if you jump, you might never come back.

It's not thrilling. It's not romantic. It's not a Netflix montage with uplifting music.

It's *paralysing*.

Your mind tells you to step back. At least 'back there' you know the rules, it says. You know what to expect. You know how to be liked. You know the world accepts this version of you, even if it doesn't feel like *you* anymore. It's safe, it's comfortable, it carries no risk.

So, the question becomes, why on earth would anyone choose to leap? Why would they walk away from certainty, security and comfort? For one simple reason: staying where they are means killing their soul.

I have come to realise that every time my mind says, "Stay where you are. Don't do that scary thing. Why would you leave the job you're good at?" that is my body screaming at me to move, and I must be willing to accept that I will feel extremely uncomfortable while I do it. I must ***do it scared.***

As Tony Robbins says, *"Change only happens when the fear of staying the same becomes greater than the fear of making the change."* **You don't leap because you're *fearless*. You leap because staying where you are becomes more painful than the fear itself.**

There comes a day when your soul refuses to shrink any further. On that day, the cost of staying small, quiet or misaligned becomes too much to bear. The truth claws its way to the surface and says, *"We either jump, or we die here."*

Only in that moment, breath caught, heart racing, hands shaking, do you realise something incredible.

The edge is not your enemy; it is your invitation.

'Okay' Is Dangerous

When life is 'okay' we don't question it. We settle, we adapt, and we tell ourselves stories like 'other people have it worse' or 'this is just how it is'. We wear our mild discontent like a badge of adulthood because 'okay' is comfortable enough to convince us to stay, even when leaving is the only way to truly live.

I've known several people who worked the same job for twenty years. They didn't hate it, but they didn't love it either. Every year, they told themselves they'd leave when it became unbearable. They would move if a certain thing stopped working or if another thing didn't change. But unbearable never came. Instead, *bearable* ate them alive, one quiet, safe day at a time, until they realised they'd traded the best years of their lives for something they never really wanted.

When things finally fall apart, when we break, when our discomfort becomes unbearable, that is when we're forced to stop pretending. That is when the truth can no longer be ignored, because it has become so much louder than our fear. Pain, real, undeniable pain, has a strange way of saving us.

If you're on the edge right now, and the storm feels violent, and the cliff face behind you is crumbling, maybe that isn't failure. Maybe that's freedom, disguised as everything falling apart. Sometimes it takes losing control of the old life to create the one that's *actually yours*.

I spent twenty-seven years trying to find something. After jumping off that edge, I found it in myself. Things had got so bad that at every new turn, I had one choice: I do this, or I die.

I didn't *want* to die. I must emphasise that. But also, I didn't want to live like this.

I was born a little girl named Jessica, with a big smile, big eyes, and I'm still pulling off the big ears, somehow! I grew up in Wigan, a working man's town in the northwest of the UK with a mindset and culture that ingrains in its people a fear of being different. When you are different in a place like this, you bury any indications that that might be the case. You suppress those thoughts and focus on any distractions you can.

I had an amazing family, and I was good at sport. I was lucky to have these advantages, and I continue to be grateful for them.

Let me tell you something, though. Wanting more isn't selfish. Staying small is.

As the years passed, the cracks widened. What I had buried started surfacing in quiet moments, in angry outbursts, in a deep exhaustion I couldn't explain. At twenty-seven, I stood on a prison landing as an experienced officer most grown men wouldn't mess with. I had begun to put both myself and my colleagues in some dangerous situations. I had run out of energy to keep living inauthentically and was angry at the world. My sense of perspective had gone out the window, and my mental health had taken such a nosedive that I had no idea of the chaos I was causing.

I had reached that edge. Not the poetic kind – the real one. The kind where your soul starts screaming louder than your fear. I had followed the script that was written for me, but inside, with a deep, bone-tired kind of emptiness, a scream without sound, I felt like a stranger to myself. My choices narrowed to one: leap or lose myself for good.

People think standing on the edge is about drama or bravery. But it's not, it's about exhaustion. Exhaustion from running, from hiding, from shaping yourself into a version of you that the world can tolerate. That's the part people don't see.

They see the leap and call it courage. But the edge? The edge is desperation. The edge when staying becomes harder than leaving, even if leaving might cost you everything.

You don't leap because it feels good. You leap because not leaping feels like a slow, invisible death. The death of your joy, your peace and your truth.

I had spent twenty-seven years pretending that 'okay' was enough and trying to be grateful for a life that was never really mine. Telling myself I could manage, that I was strong, that I should be thankful for family, for sport, for success.

But strength without authenticity is just survival.

I was tired of surviving. I had tried everything, and I could no longer live life as Jess. I didn't want to kill her; I wanted to take everything about her with me. I just couldn't have her be the image anymore. I wasn't a girl, and I knew it in my soul.

So when people ask me about transitioning, I don't say I was brave. I say it was necessary. I had already tried the alternative and lived the life that was 'safe', and it was slowly killing me.

That's what the edge feels like. It's not about wanting more. It's about no longer being able to live with less – of yourself. I had only one decision left to make. Either I transition – in a world that tells me I shouldn't – or the road ends here.

The Quiet

Silence can be deafening when you've spent your whole life drowning it out.

When the noise stops, the job, the roles, the expectations, the constant pressure to be okay, you're left with the one thing you can't escape: *yourself.*

And for most of us, that's the scariest place to be. I had spent years keeping myself busy trying to 'fix my mental health' or 'do what makes me happy'. I was always striving for something more, to achieve better, work harder and be constantly challenged mentally and physically.

At nineteen years old, I joined the Royal Air Force, which was, hands down, one of the best decisions I ever made. It provided me with all the structure, belonging and challenges I needed to keep me sane. It made me stand tall and proud, because I was part of something so much bigger than myself. Just writing these words fills my eyes with tears. I can still smell the jet fuel in the air, hear the low hum of engines on the tarmac, and feel the weight of the uniform on my shoulders. There was a pride in walking across the base that I'd never felt before, like I belonged to something solid, something that couldn't be shaken.

When I joined, as a family we all thought, "We've cracked it, this is what Jess has always needed," and it was, for approximately four years… until I stopped flying around the world for long enough to sit at a desk for five minutes. As soon as I did, there it was – every terrifying feeling, the weight of anxiety and emotion on my chest, and the sensation of dread with no idea why it was there or what it meant. I came to the realisation that I had never actually *sat with Jess*.

The quiet holds a mirror we want to avoid, and so, we fill our days with noise from devices and busyness. Neuroscience shows that our brains crave novelty and distraction when avoiding pain. Your brain isn't addicted to your phone; it's addicted to the little dopamine spike that keeps you from feeling what you're afraid to feel. The single mum who keeps the TV on 24/7 doesn't do it for the shows, but for the background voices. If the house is quiet, she will begin thinking about all she has lost.

The problem is, dopamine is a quick hit. Truth is a slow burn. One is numbing. The other is healing. That's why the scroll feels easier than the silence; the silence offers no dopamine hit, only truth. It doesn't flatter, it doesn't distract, it doesn't let us hide behind being 'busy'. It just reflects. And if we've spent years building a life that isn't truly ours, that reflection can be unbearable.

That's why we scroll, that's why we drink, that's why we work late, chase validation, stay in the wrong relationships, keep the TV on, keep the volume up. Because sitting in the quiet means meeting parts of ourselves we've tried to outrun.

We all have our own version of that noise. Where do you hide from yourself? What's your noise?

Maybe for you, it's refreshing Instagram every five minutes, or pouring another glass of wine before the conversation gets too real. Maybe it's saying yes to social plans you don't want, just so you're not alone with your own thoughts. We all have our ways of turning up the volume so we don't have to hear ourselves.

My dad has always told me, "You cannot lie to yourself." In the quiet, *you cannot lie.*

Here's what I have come to learn: as frightening as it can be, the quiet doesn't hurt you. **It heals you.**

Yes, it's uncomfortable. Yes, it uncovers every doubt, fear and insecurity you've buried. But discomfort isn't a warning sign, it's a signal that something important is trying to rise to the surface.

When I first came out to my family, I said, "I'm transitioning from Jess to Jax," and in that moment, I felt like I had just lost everything that Jess was. This ex-military, rugby-playing gay woman, this whole identity I had built over twenty-seven years – gone in an instant.

And because I had come out now, I couldn't hide behind Jess anymore. I had to be Jax, but I had no idea *how* to be Jax. I didn't know who Jax was yet. I still looked like Jess and a woman, and I still felt exactly the same, except I had thrown away everything that had protected me up to this point, along with what I thought was the soul of and the person I knew and loved.

I never thought that feeling would hit me so hard. I had spent time rehearsing it in my head, knowing I needed to do this, that I had reached breaking point and had to do the very thing I was so terrified of. Once I had done it, I thought, "I'm meant to be happy!" yet there I was, feeling more suicidal than ever before.

What I learned was crucial:

In any transition, **you must grieve the role you played.** I had to give myself time, not only to build my identity as Jax, but to grieve the version of Jess I was leaving behind. I had to give myself permission to let parts of me disappear and to take the parts I still needed to help me become who I truly was.

This is the part people miss. We are all so terrified of the changes we need to make that we forget to give ourselves the grace to process them. Don't skip this. Most people never do this work, and it's why they never feel free.

Whether you're changing careers or ending a relationship, coming out of the military or losing a parent, you must allow yourself to go through an element of grief. Say goodbye to the version of you that you were in that role: daughter, employee, partner. You must let parts of the old you go to make space. That space will feel terrifying. This is why most people avoid it and distract themselves back into the life they no longer want.

We avoid silence because we think it will break us. But what if it's the very thing that finally puts us back together? That's the irony. The thing we're most afraid of, the silence, is where all our answers live. We spend so much time running from the silence that we forget it is where the truth waits for us.

In the quiet, you begin to hear the voice that's been whispering all along, beneath the pressure, beneath the fear, beneath the performance. Your voice. The real one. The one that doesn't ask for permission to exist. This voice tells you what actually matters. It doesn't care about titles, followers, income or image – only truth. And truth, while often painful, is always freeing.

But you must sit with it. Not fix it. Not figure it out. Just *be with it.*

That is the inner work that people talk about. It involves holding the mirror up to yourself in the deafening silence and sitting in the discomfort that makes you feel more anxious and scared of your own mind than you thought possible. Do not numb it, do not turn it away, just breathe through the fear until it softens. And it *will* soften, because fear, when seen and heard, loses its power.

In the quiet, you start to realise you don't need to become someone new. You just need to come home to who you were before the world told you who to be. It's not glamorous. It's not quick. But it is the most powerful thing you'll ever do, because when you stop running from yourself, you start running towards the life that was always yours. And sometimes, running towards that life starts with nothing more than saying *no* when you'd usually say *yes*, or taking a different route home… just to remember you can.

The Climb

Can I tell you a secret? You won't like it, but bear with me.

Once you leap, there's no immediate reward. No magic waiting to catch you. No instant peace. There's just the fall... and then the ground. And then comes the long, quiet, terrifying *climb back* up. You're not where you were, but you're nowhere near where you want to be.

> *"Everyone is jealous of what you've got; no one is jealous of how you got it."*
>
> – Jimmy Carr

Everyone wants the view but not the climb. People see the trophies but not the training ground. This is the lonely chapter, the place where you don't fit in with your old friends anymore, but you don't yet have the outcomes to fit into a new group of friends. You're stuck in the space in between where everything feels unfamiliar and unstable. You're in the messy middle.

It's the month after the breakup. The texts have stopped, but the bed still feels too big. It's the first week in a new city, and you don't yet know which coffee shop makes your drink right. It's the first night in your own place, where the silence is deafening but, strangely, also full of possibility.

In the messy middle, your old life is gone, but your new one hasn't arrived yet.

It's awkward. It's lonely. It's unstable, even. But you also get to decide who walks with you to the top.

This isn't a story in which you find yourself at the summit overnight. Most people don't realise that an overnight success usually takes around ten years. Ten years of false starts. Ten years of thinking you've finally got it, only to slide back down and start again. Ten years of people asking why you haven't 'made it' yet. This is a story in which you must wake up every day and *choose yourself* again and again, without any proof that it will get easier.

It's sending the CV you've rewritten ten times. It's walking into the gym for the first time in years. It's telling your partner you're not happy. It's saying 'I'm not okay' out loud.

You do the thing. You feel the fear. You question everything. And then you do it again.

You do it scared.

For me, it was opening my mouth in a room full of people who still called me Jess. For you, it might be ordering coffee without apologising for existing. Or closing the laptop at six pm and going outside. These are not small things. These things are your training ground, and like any training ground, it's repetitive. It's heavy. You'll wonder if the training is even doing anything until one day you realise the weight you're lifting is lighter, not because it's changed, but because you did.

Do the thing anyway, even though it's scary. One of my best friends (Dani Wallace) and I are striving to do important, impactful things within the world, and so we must continue to live and work outside of our comfort zone. She calls me most days and says, *"Today's a scary one,"* and often my reply is, *"Yep, today's scary again,"* and we continue with what we need to do. We are aware that, regardless of how scary it is, we will do it anyway.

'Do it scared' has consistently been my phrase over my lifetime, and especially in the last four years since beginning my gender transition. Because the fear never really leaves, particularly in the early days. It's there when you speak your truth. It's there when you walk into a room and don't know if people will accept you. It's there when you show up as your new self, while still grieving the old one. It's there when your voice shakes, your hands tremble, and your heart feels like it's trying to climb out of your chest. It's there when the tears sit at the back of your throat and you're trying with everything you have not to run back to everything that is safe and comfortable.

I've slid backwards more times than I can count. There have been days when I swore I was done, when the climb felt like a joke, and nights when the old life whispered to me like a siren song, promising safety if I'd just turn around. And sometimes, I listened… for a while. But the next morning, I picked up the rope again.

Fear has walked beside me every step of this journey. But you know what else has?

Determination.

Not confidence, not certainty; just a quiet decision that no matter how scared I was, I would not go back to living a life that wasn't mine. I had done that already. I had played the part, I had worn the smile, I had earned the titles and followed the rules, and it nearly killed me.

So now, I do it scared.

This life is mine, I've got one shot, and it's *worth it*. I get up on the days when my mind tells me I'm not enough. I show up when the world says I should stay quiet. I take the next step, even when I can't see where it's leading. Because something inside me knows, this climb is mine.

We think we want to be dropped at the top of the mountain. We imagine how good it will feel when we get there, when we're 'fixed', when we're fearless, when we're ready, when everything makes sense. But if you didn't climb it, it won't feel like yours. You'd look around and wonder if you deserved it. Being airlifted to the top wouldn't give you pride, it would cause you doubt. You'd feel like an imposter in your own success.

But when you climb it? When you learn to enjoy the journey and understand that it is **meant to be hard – this is what hard feels like?** When you claw and fight for every step. When you cry, and shake, and stumble your way through the pain and still keep going? You *own* that summit. You prove to yourself that you are who you say you are. You build real confidence in you, and you *become* the person who belongs there.

Every hard moment, every uncertain step, every night you cried on the floor wondering if you could do this, builds something in you that can never be taken away.

If you take nothing else from this chapter, take this: you are being built, not broken.

Becoming **doesn't happen in comfort. It happens in the climb.**

One day, you will stand at the summit that you can't see yet. You'll look back and realise that every time you thought you were breaking, you were building. The future you is watching right now, silently begging you not to give up.

Right now, if you are in that place, afraid, lost, unsure: You are not broken. You are not failing. You are not weak. **You are climbing.** And the climb will make you unrecognisable to the you who almost didn't start. At some point, you have to let go of the person who got you this far, so you can become the one who takes you the rest of the way. That is how you become who you were always meant to be.

Keep going.

Do it scared.

Reflection

If you've reached your own edge, ask yourself: What's the whisper I've been ignoring? What am I pretending is 'okay' but is really eating me alive? What's one step, small or big, that would take me closer to my truth?

And then, take it.

Step onto the rock, even with the wind in your face. Grip the edge. Feel the fear. And move. Because if you wait for the storm to pass, you'll never leave the cliff. Leap scared. Climb tired. Stand shaking. Just don't stop.

You are here for more, and the climb is how you find it. So take the step. Take it even if your legs shake. Even if your voice cracks. Even if the fear screams louder than your courage. **You're not here to survive this life. You're here to own it.**

So go. Do the thing. Send the message. Quit the job. Sign the paper. Book the flight. Walk out the door. Whatever your edge is, leap. **Do it scared.**

2

THE GRACE TO GRIEVE

The Unexpected

The room was quiet, but it felt deafening. My mouth was dry, and my pulse drummed in my ears so loudly it drowned out the world. My chest was tight. My hands still shook from what I'd just done. There's a moment when your body knows something before your mind has caught up, when your breath catches in your throat and your hands won't stop trembling. At that moment, you realise you've crossed a line you can never step back over.

I'd leapt out of the old life and into the unknown. No one warns you that the bravest decision of your life might shatter you before it saves you. They tell you the leap is the hard part, but they don't say that it's the silence after, the part when the world doesn't cheer and the weight doesn't lift, and you're left carrying the ghost of the old life, that breaks you wide open.

You leap. You do the terrifying thing. You walk away from a life that was suffocating you. You stand in the quiet. You tell yourself, "I should feel free now. Is this it?"

Instead, you feel lost. You feel heavy. You feel like you've left part of yourself behind, and in a way, you have. Every change, even the ones we choose, comes with grief. And grief doesn't care whether you 'wanted' the change. It comes anyway.

The silence after change can feel unbearable, like it's never going to lift. Maybe you feel that same weight in your chest right now. I've been in that place, convinced I couldn't take another step. However, here's the good news: those moments don't last forever, even when your brain tells you they will. Also, you are not broken for feeling this way, and you are not alone in it. If you're sitting with thoughts of hurting yourself, I need you to know there is another way through. Please reach for someone you trust, or for professional help. No matter what your mind tells you in the dark, the world would not be better without you in it.

This chapter isn't just about transitioning genders. Yes, that's the doorway I came through, but I've lived many other transitions, too. I have left the military, changed careers, ended relationships, moved cities, and let go of identities that once felt like home.

Your doorway might look different. Maybe it's divorce, redundancy, sobriety, illness or recovery. Maybe it's becoming a parent or becoming an empty nester. Maybe it's losing faith or finding it. Maybe it's caring for someone you love or finally caring for yourself.

The details vary, but the inner weather is the same: the ache of letting go, the disorientation of the in-between, the quiet courage it takes to build again. If that's where you are, you belong here.

It's about walking out of the home you once built for your family and locking the door for the last time, perhaps. It's about clearing the desk you've sat at for twenty years, maybe, or driving away from the only streets you've ever known. It's about shedding an identity that once felt like your skin and finding yourself in that strange, hollow place where you're free... but not yet whole.

If you're thinking, *"That's me,"* nothing is wrong with you. You're in the waiting room between lives. It's that place where the magazines are out of date, the clock ticks too loudly, and the door to your new life hasn't opened yet.

It's not weakness. It's not regret. It's the natural process of letting go. I learned this the hardest way. And the reason I'm writing this book is so you don't have to. So that you can expect the grief and the need for patience, and not feel that you are weak when they come.

When I came out and said, *"I'm transitioning, I can't be Jess anymore,"* I thought I was ready for the freedom. I thought I was prepared for the future I was fighting so hard to claim. But I wasn't prepared for the grief.

I remember going home that night after I told my family. Everything looked exactly the same, the same sofa, the same photo frames, but it felt like I'd stepped into a stranger's life. Even my own reflection felt like it belonged to someone else. The ticking of the clock felt louder. The air seemed heavier. My skin felt too tight, like I was wearing clothes that didn't belong to me.

What I hadn't expected in that very moment was to feel like I had just lost everything that Jess was. This ex-military, rugby-playing, gay woman, this whole identity I had forged over the last twenty-seven years. Everything I was had just been thrown out the window. At the same time, I had no idea yet who Jax was. So I was stuck in the middle of not being able to hide behind Jess anymore because I was Jax now, but I still looked like Jess and nothing had changed, so who was I?

I wasn't grieving the decision; I knew it was the right one. I was grieving the life I had outgrown, the version of me I had been for so long. No one had told me to expect the grief. Maybe no one told you either. Maybe you expected relief and got emptiness instead. You didn't fail. You didn't make a mistake. You're grieving, and that means you're human.

I had to begin grieving Jess. The image. The identity. The version of me that had carried me through so much, even though she wasn't truly me. I was grieving the life that *could have been,* if the world had been different, if the journey had been easier, and if I hadn't had to fight so hard.

I was also grieving the loss of certainty, the loss of safety, and the loss of comfort. I was stepping into a life with no map, no path walked before, and no idea where to even begin. I was back on the cliff edge with a blindfold on, the ground under my feet solid one second, crumbling the next.

I couldn't see then that this wasn't failure, it was the cocoon. Like winter in the garden, everything looked dead on the surface, but underground, something was preparing to grow. The old was dissolving, but the new hadn't formed yet. It wasn't meant to feel clear; it was meant to feel lost, because I was becoming someone I hadn't met yet.

At first, I fought myself. I stood in front of the bathroom mirror, gripping the sink, whispering, *"You should be happy now. You've done the hard part. You can't fall apart now."* When you're in that middle bit, that messy, uncomfortable, awkward bit that makes you feel like every decision was the wrong one, and that's where I was then. I had no idea who I was, no idea how I was going to get through, and I felt like a complete freak. I was more suicidal than I had ever been.

But here's what I've come to learn: **You cannot heal what you refuse to grieve.**

Grieving requires grace. Not urgency to *'get over it'*. It requires sitting with the loss, honouring it, and taking everything that you love and cherish along with you in some way to form your new identity. Leave behind shame and judgement. This allows you to move through it, instead of carrying it with you like an invisible weight.

You'll move through it in your own way. For me, one way I've done this is through tattoos. On my arm, I carry two *Lion King* references: 'Remember who you are' and the 'Hakuna Matata' symbol. As a child, I must have watched that film hundreds of times, long before I knew the life lessons it was quietly teaching me. 'Remember who you are' reminds me, in the hardest times, to come back to myself. 'Hakuna Matata' reminds me to let go of the constant worry and anxiety I once carried everywhere. Those simple words from a children's movie have been a compass for me as an adult, especially through the moments when I felt completely lost.

> *One way to start: Write down the version of you you're leaving behind. Thank them for what they gave you. Then write down what you hope the next version will bring you.*

Grief Has Many Faces

It's the dad who walks past his grown son's empty bedroom, running his hand along the doorframe like it's the last thread holding him to that version of life. It's the woman who finally sells the home she built with her ex, hearing the echo of their laughter in rooms that will soon belong to strangers. It's the graduate who leaves the campus they called home for four years, realising the friendships they swore would last forever now have to survive in the real world. It's the person who walks out of their office on their last day of a career they spent decades building and suddenly doesn't know who they are without their title. It's the athlete who hangs up their jersey, the soldier who takes off their uniform, the parent who waves their youngest child off to start their own life. It's even the moment you pack away the clothes of a body you no longer live in, or delete the phone number you once knew by heart.

Different stories, same ache.

Grief isn't just for the loss of people. It shows up every time we leave a part of ourselves behind. We grieve identities. We grieve roles. We grieve friendships and communities that no longer fit. We grieve the version of life we thought we'd have. And sometimes we even grieve the version of ourselves we pretended to be, because as exhausting as it was, it still gave us a sense of place.

Think about the last time you said goodbye to a version of yourself. Maybe you didn't even realise that's what you were doing at the time. Maybe it was the day you stopped wearing a wedding ring, the day you boxed up the uniform, or the day you signed papers that changed your name. We don't always cry in those moments. Sometimes we just stand there, holding the thing that defined us, wondering how something so small can carry the weight of who we were.

Anytime we say goodbye to something, someone, or some place, we must let go of the version of ourselves we were in that situation to make room for the new version we are becoming. All the while we take the lessons we have learned and the parts of us we cherish, and we grow into who we truly are. A beautiful but painful experience, just like the butterfly.

Many people ask me why I have a big butterfly tattooed on my neck. My answer is always the same. I say, *"It represents transformation; it represents transition. We only really appreciate the beauty of a butterfly. We fail to recognise everything that butterfly had to go through to achieve something so beautiful."*

We all have our own cocoons, the places, roles and identities that feel safe but keep us small. We underestimate how much hell we must endure to break out of our own cocoon and spread our wings.

The cocoon is dark, cramped and silent, the kind of silence that hums in your ears because you've been in it too long. From the outside, it looks like nothing is happening, like you're stuck, like you've stopped growing. But inside, everything you thought you were is breaking down. Becoming isn't tidy. You lose your shape, your reference points, you feel like you're disappearing, with no proof that anything good is coming. The caterpillar doesn't simply sprout wings; it completely dissolves into a thick, shapeless soup before reforming into something entirely new. But that's the work of the cocoon, to dismantle what can't come with you, to liquefy the parts of you that kept you crawling when you were meant to fly. The darkness is not failure. It's the forge. You are not breaking down, you are breaking open.

Most people don't know this, but if you help a butterfly out of its cocoon too soon, it dies. The struggle to get free is what pumps blood into its wings. We are the same; we need to fight to make us strong enough to fly.

I wasn't just grieving Jess. I was grieving the life I'd built around her, the safety of the mask I could hide behind, the relationships that only worked when I was performing a version of myself, and the places that had brought me that first sense of real belonging, even if that belonging was conditional.

One thing really shook me throughout this process: I realised that grief and gratitude can exist at the same time. You can be grateful for your decision, and still deeply sad for what it cost you. You can love where you're going and still mourn where you've been. You can feel free and still ache for the comfort of the familiar. Grief is not proof that you've made the wrong choice. It's proof that you are human and that letting go always costs something.

Your new life will cost you your old one. Pay it gladly.

It's the most expensive thing you'll ever buy, and the only thing worth the price.

Ask yourself: What price am I paying right now? And is the future I'm building worth it?

Why We Fight Grief

You're halfway through washing the dishes when a song comes on the radio and suddenly you're standing at the sink with tears streaming down your face, hands still in the suds.

You can't outrun grief. It's faster than you. It hides in songs you thought you'd forgotten, in the smell of someone's perfume in the supermarket, in the street you haven't driven down for years. It will wait for you as long as it takes.

We fill the calendar, keep the house spotless, work late, scroll endlessly, take on one more thing, anything to avoid the moment when we sit down and realise what's gone. And yet, no matter how fast you run from it, grief always catches up, often when you least expect it.

Most of us don't know how to grieve change. We think if we're sad, it means we're failing. We think if we're hurting, we should have stayed where we were. We think if we feel lost, we were wrong to leap. So, we fight the grief. We rush to 'get over it'. We shame ourselves for not being 'better' already. We pile pressure on top of the pain. And in doing that, we stop ourselves from healing.

You cannot heal a wound you won't look at.

You can't integrate the parts of your past that you refuse to honour. You can't move forward whilst dragging invisible grief behind you. That's why grief requires *grace*.

You must let yourself feel it.

You must give yourself permission to sit in the sadness, without judgement. Cry for what was, honour what was, thank it for getting you here, and slowly, gently, start releasing it. Not because you hate it, but because you no longer need to carry it.

Grieving With Grace

It took me a long time to understand that grieving Jess didn't mean rejecting her. It didn't mean deleting everything she was. It didn't mean killing her. It meant recognising that I couldn't build a new life whilst pretending the old one hadn't mattered. Jess carried me through twenty-seven years. She fought battles too hard for me to even explain. She survived when I didn't think we would. Jess was the definition of *resilience*.

I just want to put my arms around her and thank her with all my heart for not giving up and tell her everything is going to be okay. Grieving her wasn't weakness. It was respect. It was love. It was *necessary*.

I had to let myself cry. I had to let myself miss the version of me that had been safe, even if it had been stifling. I had to let myself feel the ache of letting go. And slowly, as I did, something shifted. The sadness softened. The fear began to lift. And piece by piece, I started to build a new sense of self, not by erasing Jess, but by carrying the best of her with me into who I was becoming.

It wasn't some big breakthrough. It was in small, quiet actions of showing up, speaking up, trying again, that I slowly built the new version of me. The identity didn't come first. The doing did.

That is the grace of grief.

It's not about rejecting the past. It's about integrating it, so you can move forward lighter, freer, and more whole.

If you're in your own grief right now, whether you've left a relationship, a career, an identity, a community, a version of yourself, hear this...

You are not wrong for feeling it. You are not weak for feeling it. You are not going backwards. You are becoming. This is part of the process. When people tell you it's going to be hard but to stick with it, *this is* what hard feels like. You're in it. This is part of the process.

You are allowed to honour what was, even if you outgrew it. You are allowed to miss what was, even if you knew it couldn't sustain you. You are allowed to grieve the version of yourself who didn't know how free and happy they could be.

Grieving is not letting go of love. It's letting go of the illusion it could be the same.

Whether you're saying goodbye to a version of yourself, a person you loved, or a life you built, grief isn't rejection, it's respect.

The Gifts of Grief

Grief doesn't just change you. It grows you.

The first time I laughed after months of grief, it startled me. It felt too big for my chest, almost like my ribs couldn't contain it.

Do you know what surprised me the most?

Grief, when you give it grace, teaches you things nothing else can. It teaches you compassion, for yourself and for others. When you've sat with your own heartbreak, you understand how much everyone is carrying. You speak softer. You listen deeper. You stop expecting people to 'just get over it' because you know how long some losses live in the bones.

Grief also teaches you gratitude. It reminds you that nothing is guaranteed. It sharpens your awareness of what matters. It helps you hold joy more tenderly, because you know what it's like to live without it.

And finally, grief teaches you resilience, one of the greatest gifts you can build as a human being. Not the forced, grit your teeth kind, but the quiet strength that comes from surviving the moments you thought would break you. The kind of resilience that says, *"I can do hard things. I've done them before. And I will keep going."*

So in other words, grief, when you give it the space and grace it needs, helps us grow and become better people. Not 'better' in the glossy, perfect sense; better in the way that matters. More compassionate. More grounded. More human. The kind of 'better' that doesn't come from winning, but from losing and finding the courage to stand back up. This pain is not wasted. Every tear, every sleepless night, every moment you thought you couldn't do this, it's all shaping you into someone you will one day thank for not giving up.

Sitting With It

I wish someone had told me that you don't have to have a plan for grief. You don't have to 'do it right'. You just have to give it space. For me, it looked like letting myself cry when I needed to, no matter how inconvenient it felt. I talked to my closest people: I have found that if you can let yourself and those closest to you make fun of your biggest insecurities, no one in this world can touch you. Admit to them that you're struggling and allow them to help you by sitting in that with you.

I took quiet time, whether it was journalling, walking or sitting in my car for an extra ten minutes when everything felt too loud. I was kind to myself on the days when grief pulled me under. You must try to give yourself the same kindness as you would give others.

Some days it will feel manageable. Some days it will flatten you. Both are normal. Both are okay. Some mornings, my victory was just to get out of bed. Other mornings, it was to manage to look people in the eye whilst speaking to them. Victories seem small individually, but they add up to something stronger than you can imagine.

And with every wave you let yourself feel, you create more space for the new life to take root.

> *Grief rule: If the wave comes, ride it. Don't schedule it, don't shame it, just let it pass.*

The Next Question

The climb doesn't start when the grief ends. The climb starts here, with the weight still in your chest and the courage to take the first step anyway.

Eventually, slowly, the grief shifts.

Not because it disappears, but because you grow around it. One day, the ache eases. The sadness becomes softness, not a weight. And in that space, a new question begins to rise:

"What do I want to carry forward? And what do I need to release?"

It's a bit like losing someone you love. You must grieve the person, as well as the version of you that you were with them. In the early days, the grief is too raw for you to think about the happy memories; they just hurt. But with time, the pain softens, and you find you can hold the good moments without breaking. You can carry the joy of who they were without the heaviness of wishing things could be the same. Our old selves are like that too. Once we've grieved them properly, we can take the best of them forward without being held hostage by the past.

A friend sent me a quote recently, just when I needed to hear it, that stopped me in my tracks: "If your life was a movie and the audience were screaming at the screen for you to do something, what would they be saying? Whatever it is, do that."

When you're frozen in the fog of what to keep and what to let go, borrow the audience's voice until you can hear your own.

And now is where, in the next part of the work, it really gets interesting. You begin to choose, with intention, the pieces that will build your next chapter, because not everything from the old life belongs in the new one. Not everything in the new life will serve the person you're becoming. You start to see clearly what is truly yours, and what never was. You start to realise which parts of your old life can come forward, and which ones need to stay behind. Grief gives you the perspective to discover what to keep and what to let go.

But none of this choosing can happen if you try to rush through grief. You can't skip this part, because it's what clears the space for what comes next. The climb starts here, and if you can take a single step with grief still in your chest, you've already started winning. Every climb starts heavy. But the weight in your chest today is the proof that you're still carrying the courage that got you this far, and it will carry you the rest of the way.

You're carrying more than you should right now, but not more than you can. Keep going, because the climb isn't just about reaching the top. It's about becoming the kind of person who can keep climbing, no matter what the view looks like when you get there.

You're not climbing away from your grief. You're climbing with it, until one day, you realise it's not heavy anymore. And when you reach that place, there's a different kind of silence. Not the silence that crushes you after the leap, but the kind that fills you with peace, the quiet that tells you, "You made it."

And that is exactly where we're going next, into the climb that will test every muscle you've built, and show you exactly who you are.

3

THINGS TO KEEP, THINGS TO LOSE

REBUILDING A LIFE THAT'S FINALLY YOURS

The Inventory

Once the grief starts to soften just enough that you can breathe again, a new question arrives. Not loud, not urgent, but steady. Like a whisper that won't leave you alone…

"What do I want to bring with me?"

That's the moment when the rebuilding begins. It begins not in some dramatic montage but in the quiet decision to sort through the pieces, not all of them broken, just no longer needed, and decide what still belongs.

It's like clearing out a house you've lived in your whole life. Some things, like that old jumper that kept you warm but always itched your skin, you realise served you once but don't belong anymore. Other things you pick up and they make you smile, because they still feel like *you*. And some you hold and know instantly that they were always a little too tight, too heavy, too much about surviving, not living.

Maybe for you it's not a jumper. Maybe it's the job title, the friend group, the role in your family that you never asked for but learned to wear.

This is where the work gets surgical.

And sacred.

You ask yourself, piece by piece, "Does this still serve me? Did this ever belong to me, or was I just told I needed it? Am I keeping this because it's aligned or because it's familiar?"

Just like our physical space, our internal identity gets cluttered too. Beliefs, habits, labels and roles start stacking up until you're carrying a life that doesn't even feel like your own. And in the transition? You get a chance to put all of it down.

The Tools of Survival Aren't Meant to Build Your Future

Survival skills aren't useless, but they're not blueprints for the life you actually want.

There comes a moment when the skills that kept you alive start killing the life you want. That's the moment I faced one afternoon, like a gust of cold air that stopped me in my tracks:

What got me here can't take me there.

The qualities that helped me survive as Jess: the hyper-independence, the need to prove myself, the over functioning, the perfectionism, the 'I'm fine' mask, were all necessary in a world that didn't know who I was. They were armour. And that armour served its purpose.

Maybe you've got your own version of that armour. A 'tough guy' image you've worn at work so no one ever sees you sweat. The constant humour you use to dodge hard conversations. The busy calendar you hide behind so no one asks how you're really doing. It works, until it doesn't. One day you realise the joke isn't funny anymore, the meetings don't mean anything, and the mask you've been wearing has started to suffocate you.

Armour always has an expiry date. You can either take it off yourself or wait until life tears it off in the middle of the battlefield.

What once kept you safe will eventually keep you stuck.

Psychologists call this a loss of 'self-concept clarity', when the lines between who you truly are and who you've had to pretend to be start to blur. Research shows that low self-concept clarity is linked to higher anxiety, lower resilience, and a constant feeling of being 'off'. Clarity can't exist under armour. You have to take it off to see yourself clearly again.

When you finally reach a place of truth, that armour becomes a dead weight. The most courageous thing you can do is take it off, piece by piece, even when you feel naked without it.

It's like the corporate leader who finally walks away after twenty years in the same company. His title is practically stitched to his identity. But when he leaves, he realises the leadership skills can stay, while the belief that his worth came from a business car has to go.

I remember listening to Brené Brown talk about the difference between *fitting in* and *belonging*. Fitting in is about becoming what people need you to be. Belonging is about being who you are. One protects you. The other frees you. In my life as Jess, I had mastered fitting in. I knew exactly how to play the part that kept me accepted, praised and safe. I mean, it took the high school years of hell for me to figure it out, but we mastered it in the end. Despite this, I never once knew what it felt like to truly belong to myself.

Taking off the armour is terrifying. Maybe you've already felt this, that uncomfortable itch of knowing you've outgrown your own disguise. You wonder if anyone will still recognise you without it. The right people *will*. And when they do, you'll wonder why you wore it so long.

Keep the Fire, Drop the Mask

I think people assume that when you transition, whether it's gender, career, lifestyle or mindset, you throw everything out and start over. But that's not true. The goal isn't to burn down who you were but to keep the parts of you that were real and finally let them breathe. It's like opening a window in a house you didn't realise had gone stale. The air rushes in, and suddenly you remember what oxygen tastes like.

For me, I kept the fire. The grit. The fighter. The protector. The leadership. The humour. The sensitivity I used to think might be weakness. The weirdness I used to hide. I let go of the mask. The performance. The version of me people clapped for but never saw. The over responsibility. The hypermasculinity I'd picked up to overcompensate for feeling like I was in the wrong body.

It was like being the athlete who hangs up her jersey for the last time, not because she doesn't love the game, but because she no longer recognises the person she had to become to stay in it. She keeps the discipline, the team spirit and the drive, but leaves behind the need to prove herself through constant wins.

You don't need to become someone else. You need to become someone *real*.

So here's your challenge: make your own 'keep and drop' list today. Do this on paper. Seeing it in front of you has a way of making the decision for you.

What qualities feel like oxygen in your lungs? **Keep them.** What habits feel like a chokehold? **Drop them.**

The list doesn't need to be perfect; it just needs to be honest.

If you're not sure where to start, try this:

- Keep the part of you that feels like home.
- Lose the part that feels like a performance.
- Keep the thing you'd do for free, even if no one noticed.
- Lose the thing that drains you, even if people praise you for it.

Maybe it's keeping your love of late-night deep talks, but dropping the habit of agreeing to plans you don't want just to avoid disappointing people. Or keeping your creativity, but dropping the perfectionism that makes you never finish a project. These choices don't always happen on a mountaintop; most happen in the small, quiet moments of deciding what version of yourself you'll be today.

Letting Go of People (and the fear that comes with it)

There's something else we don't talk about enough: *Letting go of people who only loved the older version of you.*

And that doesn't mean they are bad people. It just means the relationship was built on a version of you that doesn't exist anymore. It hurts, but it's part of the climb.

There have been people in my life who couldn't make the transition with me, not because they hated me, but because they were still holding on to Jess. Some of them needed more time. Some of them never came around. I had to stop shrinking myself to keep those relationships on life support.

It's not rejection, it's realignment. You're not abandoning them, you're simply refusing to abandon yourself. If they can't love the real you, they don't get the future you. And that's not cruelty, it's clarity. You are not required to keep proving your worth to people who only ever loved the edited version of you.

That doesn't mean you need to carry hate for them. Just as they don't hate you, you don't hate them. Sometimes love has an expiry date in its current form, and letting go with grace is far more powerful than holding on with resentment.

When your growth disrupts the unspoken agreements that kept old relationships comfortable, this is called 'identity shift friction'. It's why some people pull away when you change: you're rewriting the script they were used to. And that's okay. It means you're finally living from your truth, not from someone else's expectations.

As Steven Bartlett says, "You can't become your future self while constantly justifying your past self to people committed to misunderstanding you."

'Social Identity Theory' suggests that relationships are partly built on shared identity, so when yours changes, some connections naturally fade.

Sometimes the boldest thing you can do is stop chasing people who only loved the costume. The right ones will meet you on the other side, or else they'll create new space in your life when they leave.

My dad always said this to me, and it has always stuck: *"Negative people are the biggest killers of confidence and self-esteem. Get them out your life."*

No one really prepares you for the loneliness that can follow letting go. You think clarity will immediately attract community: instead, there's a gap. You're shedding old skins and suddenly realise that you don't know who's still coming with you. That middle space is sacred, but it's rough. The nights are the hardest, when your phone stays silent, and you realise you deleted every number that only belonged to the old you. You must learn to become your own company again, before the right people find you.

You might be surprised: sometimes the people who fade and the people who stay are not those you expect. I've had people I was certain would stand by me quietly step back, and people I never imagined would understand show up with loyalty and love. That's the unpredictable part of growth: it reshuffles your circle in ways you can't always control. The ones who are meant to walk with you into your future often aren't the ones you would've bet on.

Keep the Lessons. Let Go of the Labels.

I used to wear my labels like proof I was enough.

RAF Veteran. Rugby Player. Strong Woman. Good Daughter. Tough Prison Officer.

But labels, when you outgrow them, become cages. And healing isn't just about changing how you look, it's about changing how you see yourself.

Now I hold onto the lessons, not the labels.

The discipline from the military... keep it.
The pride in physical strength... keep it.
The loyalty to my family... keep it.

But the story that I had to earn love by being useful? The belief that vulnerability made me weak? The idea that strength meant silence? **Lose it. Burn it. Leave it behind. You can keep the roots without keeping the weeds.**

Brené's TED Talk rewired me: *"Vulnerability isn't weakness, it's our more accurate measure of courage."* Amen.

Which labels do you think may have become cages for you?

The Power of Selective Memory

One of my favourite realisations came from listening to Mo Gawdat, the former Google exec turned happiness author. He said:

"We suffer not from the memory of pain, but from the story we attach to it."

Psychologists call this 'cognitive reappraisal'. It is the practice of changing the meaning you give an event so it stops holding the same emotional charge. Research from Stanford University has shown that people who consciously reframe painful experiences report lower stress levels and a stronger sense of meaning in their lives. In other words, the past doesn't change, but the power it has over you does.

That hit me like a punch to the chest. There were so many parts of my past I kept revisiting with shame, until I realised I could revisit them with compassion instead.

You don't need to forget who you were. You need to reframe your story.

Jess wasn't weak; she was surviving. Jess didn't fail; she carried me as far as she could. Jess wasn't the end of me; she was the beginning.

I never want to think of Jess as being dead. I have always tried to take everything about her with me and form my new identity as Jax. Jess was twenty-seven years of my life, and I never want her or those memories and experiences to disappear. I don't believe that is a healthy way to move forward through something so transformative. In my experience, I believe you have to do the inner work we are talking about in this book in order to truly heal and become the person you truly are.

The Cost of Comfort

There were nights I nearly retreated. Days I believed I would never be able to make it through this. I scrolled old photos, wondering if life had truly been 'that bad', and if I had made a huge mistake even trying to turn this into reality. Familiar pain felt safer than foreign peace.

But comfort isn't the same as peace. Comfort kept me alive; peace lets me live. The cost of authenticity is your comfort, and once you taste freedom, no amount of comfort is worth going back.

Chris Williamson said something once that hit me like a slap in the face:

> "Life usually has to get significantly worse before people change, because 'okay' is deceptively manageable."

He compared it to walking to the shop.

If the shop is two hundred metres away, you might think, "Eh, I'll drive later." But if the shop is ten miles away and you desperately need food, you move.

It's the same with life. When things are fine, we endure. When things are terrible, we act.

That's why 'fine' is so dangerous. It doesn't demand a breakthrough. It's just uncomfortable enough to keep you stuck but not painful enough to force your hand. It lulls you into staying small.

Psychologists call this the 'status quo bias'. Our brains have a tendency to stick with what's familiar, even when it's hurting us. Studies show we're far more motivated to escape intense pain than mild discomfort, which is why rock-bottom often triggers change, but 'fine' keeps us quietly stuck for decades.

So if your life is falling apart right now, if you're in the chaos, the heartbreak, the confusion, I know it feels awful. But maybe, just maybe, that collapse is your invitation.

Because pain moves us. *Okay* doesn't. *Okay* is the quiet killer of dreams. *Okay* will sing you a lullaby until the years are gone. Pain will kick your door in.

Okay doesn't set off alarms. It whispers, "This is fine," until you can't remember the last time you felt alive. It's the slow leak in the tyre; you don't notice you've stopped moving until the whole car is sitting on its rims. And by the time you realise, years have passed, and the life you were meant to live is parked somewhere you can't see from here. Don't wait for the flat tyre, start walking now.

Integration Over Erasure

You don't have to destroy your old self to become your true self. You just have to stop pretending that's all you are.

I still have photos of Jess everywhere: in my parents' house, on my social media, in my wallet. I do this not to cling to her, but to honour her. Integration means recognising she's part of my DNA, even if she's no longer the face on the badge.

You're Allowed to Keep Changing

Here's your permission slip: **You do not have to 'arrive'.**

There's no hurry. There's no prize for deciding on one single plan and sticking to it forever. You are not signing a lifelong contract with the version of you that exists today. You get to pivot. You get to change your mind. You get to evolve as many times as you need. The pressure to 'figure it all out' is a lie; your only job is to keep becoming more you.

I'm still learning to trust on good days. I still have moments of grief out of nowhere. And that's okay for you, too. You can be a masterpiece and a work in progress at the same time.

There's no finish line where someone hands you a medal and says, "You've arrived." You're The version of you that feels right today is allowed to be temporary. In fact, it's supposed to be. allowed to unpack and rearrange as often as you need.

Rebuilding on Purpose

If you're currently in your own version of this in-between, whether you've just left a relationship, walked away from a job, come out, transitioned, quit drinking, changed cities, or finally said 'no more' to the thing that was killing your joy, I want you to ask yourself these three questions:

1. What parts of me feel like home?
2. What parts feel like armour I no longer need?
3. Who am I without the roles I used to play?

You will not get perfect answers right away, but by asking the question, you begin the rebuild.

Your life starts becoming yours, not because of what you gain, but because of what you choose to carry forward. Freedom isn't found in becoming someone new. It's found in finally becoming yourself.

The Sorting Table

Soon I found myself laying everything out, like evidence on a detective's desk. Put it all on your own sorting table and decide, piece by piece, what stays and what goes. This isn't just my process. It's yours too. Lay out everything about yourself: your beliefs, your habits, your roles, your relationships, and see them clearly for what they are.

Do it tonight. Ten minutes. Write down everything you're carrying: roles, habits, relationships, and ask yourself, "Keep or let go?" That's it. Don't overthink it. The clarity will surprise you.

My sorting sounds like this:

> Core values I refuse to compromise… **keep.**
> Habits that only exist to please other people… **lose.**
> People who challenge me to grow… **keep.**
> Self-talk that shrinks me… **lose.**

And here's the best part: the moment you put something in the 'let go' pile, you start breathing lighter. It's instant proof you're building a life that fits.

Think of the woman who packed up the house after her divorce. She kept the Sunday morning pancakes, the holiday traditions, and the love for gardening. But she let go of the unspoken rule that her needs always came last.

You can lay out everything about you on your own sorting table. That sorting never ends, but the first pass is the hardest. And once you do it, something shifts: life stops happening *to* you and starts getting built *by* you.

> I get to choose what stays.
> I get to release what no longer serves me.
> I am allowed to evolve.
> I am allowed to keep growing.
> I don't need permission to become more me.
> And neither do you.

Your sorting table is never a one-time event. It's a lifelong practice of saying yes to what lights you up and no to what weighs you down, until one day you look around and realise, this life fits me, because I built it for me.

You don't arrive at a perfect, finished self. You arrive at a life that feels like home. Because a life that fits isn't luck. It's the result of choosing yourself, over and over, until it's impossible to imagine being anyone else.

4

THE QUIET

WHEN THE NOISE STOPS, THE TRUTH BEGINS TO SPEAK

There comes a point in every transformation when the noise fades, not because life gets easy, but because it gets real. The distractions thin out. The old habits fall away. The people who once filled the silence have stopped calling. You've cleared out the clutter, taken off the armour, and shone light on the false stories. And what's left?

You. No music. No scrolling. No performance. No audience. Just… you.

You stand under a spotlight with nowhere to run. It's that moment in a room full of people where everyone else's laughter fades, and you suddenly hear your own breath too loudly. That moment, the one most people spend their whole lives avoiding, is when everything begins.

But let's be honest: sitting with yourself is terrifying. I used to think rock bottom was losing my job, or losing my identity, or the panic attacks, or even standing on the edge, thinking, *I can't do this anymore.* That wasn't rock bottom. The real rock bottom was when the noise finally stopped, and I had to face myself. No more performing. No more pretending. No more being busy fixing, chasing, explaining, proving. Just… silence. And inside it, every part of me I had been running from.

The quiet doesn't clap. It doesn't reassure. It just hands you the truth and waits to see if you can hold it. And if you drop it? You have to pick it back up.

The Mirror of Silence

Silence is a mirror. The kind in bad hotel bathrooms, offering a harsh light and no angle to hide. It shows you the bits you've been ignoring. And that's why we run from it.

Psychologists call this 'self-confrontation,' the uncomfortable art of sitting with your thoughts without a single escape hatch. And there's a reason it feels so intense. Science says that when you first stop the noise, your brain literally thinks it's in danger. It can't tell the difference between a lion in the room and a hard conversation in your head. *Of course* it feels dangerous; your nervous system is just trying to protect you. It's like your brain is running through its emergency contact list, but really, all you did was sit on the sofa without your phone. This, by the way, is how you know things have got bad, when your brain treats 'no phone' like an actual hostage situation. Your body isn't wrong. It's doing its job. But the 'danger' isn't real. It's just you, finally sitting still long enough to notice what's been there the whole time.

In every conversation I have with someone who wants to change something in their life, whether that is a prisoner wanting to stop taking drugs, someone struggling to accept their identity, or someone who repeatedly self-sabotages their relationships, the first thing I say to them is that they need to find the courage from somewhere to look themselves in the mirror. You cannot lie to yourself, ever.

That is what silence proves to you every single time. You can't tell yourself, "It's fine," when your body says it's not. You can't pretend you're happy when your chest is tight every morning. You can't fake confidence when your thoughts are screaming doubt.

Robin Sharma says, *"You'll never rise higher than your self-identity,"* but most of us don't even know who that self is, because we've never shut the world up long enough to listen to them. Silence *makes* you look in the mirror. It doesn't flatter. It doesn't filter. It doesn't lie.

But… and here's the part no one tells you: It doesn't hate you either. It just tells you the truth.

How We Avoid Ourselves

We all have our ways of avoiding the mirror. We scroll. We drink. We binge. We hustle. We listen to ten hours of motivational podcasts but never sit still for ten minutes with our own thoughts.

Neuroscientists have found something wild: your brain reacts to these little avoidance habits the same way it reacts to addictive substances. That endless scroll? That internal need to just keep busy? It's giving you a dopamine hit. Your brain's not saying, "I'm happy," it's saying, "Thanks for the sugar rush." And then it crashes. That's why it feels easier to scroll TikTok at midnight than to sit in the dark with your thoughts. The quick hit wins, even though you always wake up emptier than before. I have done it myself. I'm fully aware that I've done that thing where you scroll until your phone drops on your face. Olympic level avoidance.

I used to call it 'being productive'. But really? I was just afraid of being still. I want you to know something that I must still tell myself often: you're not tired, you're unfulfilled. I convince myself sometimes that I'm tired from doing too much, when in reality, I'm tired of avoiding what needs my attention: myself. You might be in that exact place today, reading this, pretending it's not you.

Silence used to feel so dangerous and still does at times. It stripped away the performance I used to hide behind. And when your whole life has been a performance, even a well-meaning one, taking off the mask feels like dying.

But what I've learned is this: Silence won't kill you. Avoiding it will.

You can outrun almost anything, except yourself. One day, your legs give out, and there you are, staring at the thing you've been sprinting from.

You Can't Heal What You Won't Face

When I was living as Jess, I was 'doing the work'. At least, I thought I was. Fitness, routine, journaling, and reading every book I could find on personal growth. I thought: *If I just fix enough stuff, I'll feel better.* But healing doesn't come from fixing. It comes from listening, and from looking straight at yourself.

Peace is not being passive. The silence isn't the absence of life; it's the space where life gets heard. But you don't hear that peace in your first week of quiet. At first, all you hear is the noise you've been ignoring. You hear the grief, the shame, the fear and the parts of you that you abandoned just to survive. And yet, that's where healing begins. Not in 'moving on', but in finally sitting with what's waiting to be seen.

Avoidance isn't a rest. It's self-abandonment in disguise.

Where have you been calling it 'rest' when really you've just been running? Be honest. You thought of something just then, didn't you? It is that one thing you keep putting back in the drawer.

The Ego Fights the Quiet

In Jungian psychology, the 'ego' isn't arrogance; it's the constructed identity you believe you are. Silence threatens it because stillness forces a confrontation with your 'shadow self', the parts of you you've rejected or hidden in order to be accepted by others. This is why the ego resists: it senses that if you face those parts, you might dismantle the very identity it's worked to protect.

The ego hates silence, because silence doesn't care about titles. It doesn't care how many people liked your post. It definitely doesn't care how much you earn, how fit you are, or how clean your morning routine is. It only cares about one thing: **Are you being real?**

Jay Shetty said something once that stayed with me: *"We're so busy trying to be liked by others, we forget to like ourselves."*

In the quiet, that hits harder, because you start to realise how much of your identity was built for other people. You didn't become the strong one for yourself. You became them because someone needed you to be. You didn't become the funny one just for joy. You did it because laughter made people comfortable. And here's the hardest part: you might not like what you find in the silence at first. But don't confuse discomfort with danger. Silence doesn't punish you; it invites you. You also might find out you're funnier, braver, and way more interesting than you gave yourself credit for, so it's not all doom and gloom in there.

It says: *Come home.*

But coming home means opening doors you've nailed shut. And you know exactly which doors I mean. The thing is, you don't get to control what's behind them. And if you don't open them, you'll keep living as a guest in your own life: polite, careful, never truly putting your feet up.

The Ritual of Sitting Still

"Silence doesn't mean nothing's happening. It means something sacred is."

We live in a culture that treats stillness like failure. If you're not working, you're lazy. If you're not posting, you're irrelevant. If you're not replying instantly, you're distant. And if you're just… sitting there? You're wasting time.

I am still guilty of falling into all these traps to this day. I beat myself up for not working hard enough, not doing enough, not making enough progress.

But stillness isn't laziness. Stillness is presence. Stillness is sacred. And for a long time, I didn't know how to do it. I could train hard, lead others, even give talks on growth and mental health, but I couldn't sit still with myself without reaching for a distraction within two minutes. My biggest fear has always been my own mind. *I was petrified of the silence.* Which is pretty ridiculous, really, because my mind is awful at multitasking. Half the time, it forgets why I even walked into a room!

Stillness felt like being locked in a tiny room with a stranger who knew every secret I'd ever tried to bury. They were a version of me I didn't fully trust yet. For me, that room had piles of unanswered texts, old photos I couldn't look at, and a thousand unfinished 'I'll deal with it laters'.

But this is the lesson: if you can't sit in stillness with yourself, you're not living; you're just performing. I had to build a new kind of ritual of sitting in the silence. It is easier said than done, and one that I still have to practise every day and fight against the urge to run away from. It is not about fixing or doing or achieving. It simply allows me to be.

The Mind Isn't the Enemy

At first, silence brings chaos. Thoughts race. Regret pops up. Shame starts whispering. Fear returns. You think, *maybe I was better off busy.*

But your mind is a tool, and like any tool, it gets louder when it's left untrained. Your mind isn't punishing you. It's just finally being given airtime. You've spent years filling every gap with noise. So the first few days, maybe weeks, feel like withdrawal. But beneath the noise, you'll find clarity. And clarity isn't lightning; it's a slow unfolding.

The more you sit, the more your thoughts stop shouting. And beneath the noise, you start to feel the truth. Not the story.

Not the mask. Not the version of you you've rehearsed. But the quiet, grounded voice that says: "This is who I am. And I've been here all along."

You're Not Broken. You're Just Unheard.

We treat discomfort like danger. But discomfort is a sign that something is waking up. When I finally let Jess go and stepped into Jax, I thought everything would click. Instead, the quiet nearly broke me. But in that silence, something extraordinary happened: for the first time in my life, I started to listen without judgement. I stopped analysing every feeling. I stopped labelling thoughts as wrong or right. I just… listened.

And what I heard in the silence was this: You're not broken. *You're just unheard.* The voice, that knowing, had been drowned out for so long. And when it finally spoke, it didn't shout. It didn't scold. It whispered, *"You're safe now; you can come home."*

Your Truth Lives in the Stillness

The tattoo on my right hand reads: **Remember Who You Are**

I have always tried to live by this. On the surface, it is a quote I first heard at the age of five, rewatching *The Lion King* twenty-three times in a row. It has helped me get through everything I didn't think I would.

But underneath the surface lies what it really stands for. People think finding yourself is about discovery. Like there's a map, and one day you'll stumble on it. But it's not like that. Finding yourself is about remembering. It's about stripping away every expectation, every label, every lie the world told you to survive, until what's left is something solid. Quiet. True. And the only place you can hear that truth is in the quiet stillness.

The most important conversation you'll ever have is the one you stop running from.

The Voice You've Been Avoiding

In the chaos, there are a thousand voices: parents, bosses, coaches, friends, followers, algorithms. You ask, "What do they want from me?" "What will they think?" "Who do I need to be to belong?"

But in the quiet? There's only one voice. Yours. And at first, it doesn't even sound like yours. It sounds small. Unsure. Fragile. You question it. You think: *This can't be it… this voice is too soft to build a life on.*

But that softness? That's the point. It's soft because it's honest. And truth doesn't shout. It waits.

The voice you ignore will eventually become the life you regret.

Self-Trust Begins in Solitude

I remember once reading: *"You can't hear your purpose in a crowd."*

I think that is true of self-trust, too. You can't trust yourself if you've never been alone with yourself. You can't know who you are if you've never spent time in the raw, unfiltered company of your own being. Self-trust is not built on performance. It's built in privacy. It's built in the work nobody sees.

You can fake a lot of things in public: confidence, clarity, and even happiness, but solitude doesn't buy it.

Psychology backs this up. A theory called 'self-determination theory' says we need three things to thrive, and one of them is autonomy. In plain English, that is about doing what matters to you, not just what gets a round of applause. Think less 'standing ovation', more 'sleeping like you actually like yourself'.

You can't know what matters until you've spent enough time with yourself to find out. When you do this, you begin to realise something powerful: You don't need one hundred people to validate your direction. You don't need everyone to understand the path you're on. You just need the single voice inside to get louder than the noise outside. And that happens in the quiet. That happens when you finally become still enough to hear it. Yes, it's awkward at first, like trying to make small talk with yourself in a lift, but it gets easier.

People ask me all the time how I deal with negativity online… the trolls, the hate, the abuse. Doing this work in the quiet is so vital because you need to understand every corner of your soul, and that is no easy task. But the more you do it, the more trust and confidence you build. When I receive comments online, I can react in one of two ways: I can ignore, or I can appreciate, but I try never to take it in.

Of course, I can be incredibly grateful and appreciative of any love and support I may receive, but it does not define who I am. If you allow your self-worth to be dependent on other people's opinions, it will fluctuate depending on what someone has said to you that day. If you let the praise in, you have to let the criticism in too, and that's a dangerous game. You cannot have one without the other. If I allowed this, every time I received a negative comment, it would chip away at my self-confidence because I would have become reliant on other people's opinions about who I am as a person.

Doing this deep inner work, in the silence of your own mind, allows you to figure out and know exactly who you are, know your soul and be proud of that, no matter what. If you can master this, no one's opinion will shake that.

There's No Applause in Solitude

"The time you feel like doing it the least is when you need it the most."

– Robin Sharma

That's the quiet. That's showing up for yourself when no one's clapping, no one's watching, and you're not even sure if it's working. But that's when it counts, because when no one's watching, the mask drops. And that's when the real work begins, not changing yourself, but *meeting* yourself.

The Day I Heard the Real Me

I'll never forget one particular day; it was around six months after coming out. I was walking alone into the prison for a shift, no headphones, no talking, nothing but the sound of my feet and my breath. For the first time, the sound wasn't drowned out by the noise of proving myself. That's when it hit me, I wasn't doing anything. I wasn't performing. I wasn't fixing. I wasn't surviving. I was just *being*. And for the first time… I didn't hate who I was being with. I wasn't running. I wasn't resisting. I felt raw and a little shaky, but real.

For once, my own company didn't feel like a threat.

That was the day I realised I was finally letting the truth speak. I wasn't trying to become someone new. I was finding the truth I'd buried beneath performance, perfection, and protection for nearly three decades. I realised there and then that this was it, this was the journey, and I was finally present enough to appreciate it.

That's what silence gives you. Not fireworks. Not clarity in a sentence. But a slow, patient invitation back to yourself.

Truth Doesn't Need to Convince You

Truth doesn't argue or sell itself to you. It doesn't beg you to listen. It just waits. There's no noise left to distract you from the knowing inside you. This is why, in the stillness, so many people panic. The knowing says, "You're not happy here; you're pretending again; you already know what needs to change."

If you're honest, you've known for a while what needs to change, haven't you? We always know. We just hope we're wrong. I know what it's like to feel that knot in your stomach. That knot isn't fear, it's recognition.

When I came back from my military tour in 2017 at the age of twenty-four, I sat down with my mum and said, "Is it because I want to be a boy? Is that why I'm so depressed, mum?"

To this day, I could not tell you where in my mind that question came from. I didn't even know it was possible to transition at this point. But there was a niggle in my mind that made me ask it of the person I trust more than anyone in this world.

My mum replied, "No, of course not. You're this beautiful, athletic, amazing woman. You wouldn't be you if you weren't Jess."

In that moment, that is what we both believed. My mum tells me now that if she'd said, *"Yes Jess, you should be a boy,"* and I'd thought, *"Right, okay, I'll do it because my mum said it."* ... and then it ended up being the wrong decision, she would never have forgiven herself. And so we both buried it there and then, and I continued into my prison service career for two years before it finally hit me.

When it did, it was like the universe had been knocking on my door for years saying, **"You're going to have to deal with this at some point."**

And that's terrifying. Because once you hear it, you can't un-hear it. You can try to forget it, but it never really goes away. It becomes a whisper that shows up in every quiet moment. And eventually you must answer it.

But What If You Don't Like What You Hear?

This is the fear most people carry, even if they never say it out loud. They're not afraid of silence. They're afraid of what they'll find in the silence. What if they've made too many mistakes? What if they realise they've wasted years? What if they're not as strong as they pretend to be?

Here's what I want to say to that version of you: The truth doesn't punish. It frees. It doesn't show up to shame you. It shows up to liberate you. Whatever you find in the stillness is already there. You're not creating it, you're meeting it. And once it's seen, it loses power. Because the real fear is never the truth itself, it's the loneliness of carrying it alone.

Sharing your truth with yourself is the first act of trust. You can't expect anyone else to hold it if you won't. And the moment you see it, name it, breathe through it, you're no longer alone with it. You're home.

Therapists will tell you the danger isn't the thought itself, it's the meaning you pin on it. The label you slap on it. That's what hurts. In the quiet, those thoughts show up naked. And if you stop rushing to dress them as 'bad' or 'wrong', you realise they're just… thoughts.

The Fear of the Real You

You've done the silence. You've heard the voice. And now comes the hardest part: **Do you trust what it's telling you?**

Most people don't run from stillness because they're weak. They run because they know what lives there, and they're not sure they're ready to deal with it. If the real you steps forward, the version that doesn't perform, doesn't shrink, doesn't apologise for being different, then some relationships won't survive. Some careers won't fit. Some expectations will crumble.

And that's terrifying.

So we run back. Back to busy. Back to being liked. Back to knowing the rules. We can't sit in it for long enough to reach the other side because the uncertainty cripples us.

Some people fear failure. I feared being seen.

Here's the raw truth: Most people aren't afraid of failure. They're afraid of becoming someone they can no longer hide from. Once you meet them, you can't go back to pretending you don't know they exist.

It's why we sabotage our own growth. We drink when things get real. We scroll when the emotion rises. We go back to the person, the habit, the role we *already know* hurts us. Discomfort is familiar. Clarity demands change.

I know that you just pictured the change you've been avoiding. Don't worry, you're not alone in that. That's usually the point a person either closes the book or throws it across the room. That is fine, just pick it up again. I promise I'm not here to ruin your life.

Letting Go of the Performed Self

At some point, you have to ask: *Who am I when no one's watching?*

That question shattered me. For so long, I was only comfortable being the version of myself I thought other people needed. Jess was 'strong'. Jess was 'funny'. Jess was 'always happy'. Even when I was dying inside.

Have you ever considered what version of yourself you believe you need to be for other people? If you haven't, I encourage you to try it and ask yourself if this is the real you, or if a different version needs to exist instead. The person you're afraid to be… might just be the person you've always been. You've just never been safe enough to let them exist.

And when you've spent years becoming the perfect version of someone you're not, letting that version go can feel like death. But it's not death, it's a return.

Safety isn't the absence of risk; it's the presence of truth.

Becoming Whole, Not Perfect

This is where most of us get stuck. We finally start hearing our voice. We start imagining a life built on truth. And then fear kicks in: *But I'm not ready. I'm not healed. I'm not fixed.*

You don't have to be healed to be honest. You don't have to be fixed to be free. You just have to stop abandoning yourself. That's the quiet contract: I won't leave myself, even when I'm messy, uncertain and unfinished.

> *"You don't need to believe in yourself to start. You just need to stop believing the lies that say you can't."*
>
> **– Mel Robbins**

You are not broken. You are becoming. And becoming doesn't look like confidence. It looks like courage in motion – trembling voice, shaking hands and honest eyes.

Not fake-it-till-you-make-it…

FEEL IT TILL YOU FREE IT. That's what real self-love is. Not a Pinterest quote. Not a mirror affirmation. It's staying with yourself, even on the days you'd rather be anyone else.

You don't need perfect confidence. You need imperfect loyalty to yourself.

The Whisper You Can Trust

By now, the noise has faded. And maybe, if you've stayed long enough in the quiet, you'll begin to feel it. It is a whisper, not loud, but steady. Not urgent, but clear.

It doesn't say, "You've arrived."

It says: "You're here now. You're real. You're ready to climb back up."

The climb won't be loud either. It'll be steady, deliberate, and yours. It won't always look like fireworks or breakthroughs. Most of the time, it'll look like choosing the harder thing on a Tuesday afternoon when nobody's watching. It'll look like small, consistent steps that feel almost invisible in the moment, but which, over time, will build a life you can stand on. And the best part? No one else gets to own it, perform it, or decide it for you. It doesn't need an audience. It just needs you, showing up, one step after the other. That's where the real transformation happens: in the climb you commit to when the world isn't clapping.

The Work Beneath the Quiet

If you've made it this far, you've already done something most people never do: you've stayed.

You've stayed with the discomfort. With the silence. With yourself. But the quiet isn't just a pause. It's an invitation. So before you move on, take five minutes. No music. No scrolling. No one watching. Just you.

Ask:

> *What do I hear in the silence that I've been avoiding?*
> *What part of me have I been performing instead of protecting?*
> *What if the version of me I'm scared to meet… is actually the real me waiting to lead?*

You don't need to answer perfectly. You just need to start asking honestly. The quiet is where the truth speaks, and if you listen long enough, you'll realise it was **always your voice.**

> *"Ask yourself the questions you are terrified to answer, and you will find the road to true happiness."*
>
> **– Jaxon Feeley**

And when you finally answer, the quiet doesn't get louder. *You* do. And once you've heard yourself, you'll never again be able to pretend you can't.

There's no going back… which is kind of the point, really. Like finding out your favourite takeaway does delivery, you can't unknow it.

5

THE CLIMB

BECOMING THE PERSON WHO BELONGS AT THE SUMMIT

The Brutal Truth About Leaping

Here's the part no one tells you. After the leap, after the silence, after the moment you finally stop lying to yourself... **nothing magical happens.**

There's no fanfare. No immediate clarity. No sudden wave of confidence. There's just the fall and then the landing. Hard. Quiet. Unremarkable. And then?

The climb.

It's not a Netflix montage. Not a motivational reel. Just you, sweating, doubting, crawling your way up from rock bottom. Most people turn back, not because they're weak but because this part feels *so goddamn long.*

The In-Between Is Where Most People Quit

The in-between is brutal. You're no longer who you were, but not yet who you're becoming. You don't belong in the old room, but you haven't earned your way into the new one. Your old friends don't get it, and your new ones don't know you yet. You are stuck in the most honest place in the world:

Becoming.

It's awkward, lonely and confusing as hell. It makes you question every decision you've made and makes every bone in your body scream, "Run back to your comfort zone."

This is where the magic actually happens. Even if it feels nothing like magic right now.

There's a quote I have heard many times: "Your new life is going to cost you your old one." But what no one talks about is how *it might take a while before your new life even shows up.*

The Messy Middle Builds the Real You

> *"Everyone is jealous of what you've got, no one is jealous of how you got it."*
>
> **– Jimmy Carr**

You want to know what no one envies? The nights you cried into a pillow, wondering if this whole thing was a mistake. The days you showed up to the gym or the job or the mirror, with nothing but grit and a decision not to quit. The awkward conversations, the voice cracks, the uncertain steps forward.

That's the stuff no one claps for. But that's the stuff that builds the real you.

It's the single mum retraining at night while the kids sleep. It's the guy learning to walk again after an accident. It's the student showing up for class with yesterday's panic attack still in their chest. Robin Sharma calls it the 'pain of growth' – the internal breakdown required to reach your next level. It is not a breakdown that destroys you, but a breakdown that *rebuilds* you.

A few days before I left to join the RAF at nineteen, my mum and I were driving together when Miley Cyrus' *The Climb* came on the radio. We didn't say a word, we just sat there listening, both with tears in our eyes. For the two years leading up to that moment, I had been struggling with crippling anxiety, not knowing who I was, where I belonged, battling suicidal thoughts and the weight of just making it through each day. I know my mum had worried whether I'd even make it to the RAF at all. But deep down, in that way mothers just know, she sensed that if I did, it would be the making of me. And she was right; it saved my life.

Listening to those lyrics that day, we both knew I was standing at the bottom of my next climb. It was frightening but exciting. And the thing about climbs is, they don't stop. Every time you finish one, life eventually hands you another. You don't climb because it's beautiful. You climb because what's behind you is no longer an option.

Even now, twelve years later, my mum still teases me about how I deliberately choose challenges that will test me to my core. Just recently, when I told her about taking myself to Spain for a week-long dopamine detox to finish writing this book, she laughed and said, "Jax, I'm sure you just think, right, I'll do this now and see if that will break me."

And she's not wrong. Every climb has felt that way: scary, uncertain, but those are the climbs that have shaped me the most.

Discipline Over Motivation

Motivation is great, until it disappears. That's why discipline has to become your best mate on this climb. There were so many days I didn't feel 'brave'. Didn't feel 'authentic'. Didn't feel *anything* but tired, scared and sick of trying. But I kept going. Not because I was inspired. But because I'd already lived the alternative of the numbness, the survival and the life that didn't belong to me, and I refused to go back.

> *"You don't rise to the level of your goals. You fall to the level of your systems."*
>
> **– James Clear, Atomic Habits**

If you want to become the person who belongs at the top, build the habits now that future-you depends on. Show up even when it sucks. Rest when needed, but don't disappear.

Do it scared. Do it tired. Do it anyway.

One day, you'll thank the version of you who did.

Be Careful Who You Take Advice From

There's a moment on the climb when the doubt creeps back in. And suddenly, *everyone's voice gets louder.* People from the old life start offering opinions, not because they understand where you're going, but because they're uncomfortable with where you're headed.

"Why would you leave that job?"
"You're not the same anymore."
"You've changed."

Damn right I have. And here's what I've learned:

Never take criticism from someone who would never dare to do what you're doing.

Their comfort zone is not your home. I have heard Chris Williamson talk a lot about this on his podcast, *Modern Wisdom*. He says, *"People won't always resist your change because it's wrong. They'll resist it because it's a mirror showing them where they've stayed still."*

Your growth exposes what others have buried. Some people will hate you for digging up what they've spent years covering. Don't let their discomfort become your compass. Take advice from people on the same path, the ones doing the work, not just talking about it. The ones who've made it through their own messy middle and are still humble enough to keep climbing.

The Myth of Arrival

Here's the other lie that nearly broke me: *"One day it will all feel easy. One day I'll arrive."*

Spoiler alert: there is no summit where life gets tied in a neat little bow.

Even now, as Jax – five years into transitioning, speaking on stages, impacting lives – I still have days when I wake up and wonder what the hell I'm doing. The people who win are not the ones who feel confident. They're the ones who act anyway.

The climb never ends, because the view keeps changing. That's the best and worst part of it. You don't arrive. You evolve. And every version of you unlocks a new mountain to climb. The goal isn't to stop climbing. The goal is to fall in love with the process.

Becoming the Person Who Belongs at the Top

This might be hard to hear:

You don't build confidence by thinking. You build it by doing.

I met an individual whilst speaking at an event last week. They approached me and asked: *"How do you become so confident in speaking in front of people and telling your story?"*

I said to them what I would always say in response to a question about confidence. You have to remember that we all start sh*t. You were really rubbish at walking when you first started learning how to walk. Riding a bike? Awful! Tying your shoelaces? It took me ages!

We only build confidence by doing the reps in the gym. Laying the pieces of paper when writing a book. Chipping away at the marble to reveal the masterpiece.

You become proud of yourself by earning your own respect and by proving to yourself that you are who you say you are. It's not about how you look. It's not about external validation. It's about knowing, deep in your bones, *I showed up for me today*, even when it was uncomfortable. Especially when it was uncomfortable.

> *"You are never going to feel like it. So stop waiting to feel ready, and start building evidence that you can do hard things."*
>
> **– Mel Robbins**

That is the climb. It's just you, standing in your own vulnerability and struggle, finding the courage to try even when you don't have a clue what the outcome will be.

Show up for therapy. Say no when your body says no. Be the first to raise your hand. Ask for help. Go to the gym even if you only last ten minutes. Choose the higher path when no one's watching.

Every step is a vote for the person you are becoming.

Psychologists call this 'self-signalling'. Every action becomes evidence your brain uses to decide who you are.

Let the Work Speak

When I was in the thick of transition, I didn't know how to introduce myself. I didn't know if people saw Jess or Jax. I didn't know if I could carry this new version of me with confidence yet. So instead of proving myself, I just kept showing up and doing the work.

I would arrive outside a family party, knowing there were so many people all in one room who had never met me as Jax yet. I can feel the fear in my bones now just talking about it. Everything in me told me to just go home and not bother. But what would that achieve? I was living my truth for me; I didn't need anyone else's approval. And the more I was uncomfortable, the more it would make everyone else uncomfortable. So I used to remind myself that the more relaxed I was, the more relaxed everyone else would be. That mindset allowed me to walk into every room, own my decisions and own who I was.

I look at that version of me now and have no idea how I plucked up so much courage to do what I did repeatedly. But when you break it down, I was just doing the work, climbing, every second of the day, just doing it scared.

That's what the climb demands. Not noise. Not announcements. Not explaining yourself over and over again. Just showing up, letting the work speak, and letting the *consistency* speak. Like the artist painting in a cold garage every night for a decade before anyone buys a single piece, the climb looks different for everyone, but the work is always invisible at first. It's the least glamorous part, and the most important.

Eventually, the world catches up. But you don't need it to, because *you've already caught up to yourself.*

The Rambo Lesson

I saw this as one of the hardest two weeks of my life, and it wasn't about me. It was about my dog, Rambo. Yes, she's a girl, and yes, she absolutely rocks the name. She's a Weimaraner, a machine, hard as nails. But when she was two years old, she almost died.

One night, she became violently ill, coughing up foam and unable to keep anything down. By the time I got her to the emergency vets, she was severely dehydrated and put straight into intensive care. Over the next ten days, she got worse, with fluid on her lungs, unable to breathe without oxygen for more than fifteen minutes, and refusing food.

But here's what got me: whenever she went outside for a quick toilet break, she still tried to chase leaves, like she always had. Even in that state, she had fight in her. She wasn't ready to go.

The vet bill had hit £20,000. I told them I'd sell my house if I had to. And on day ten, the vets warned me that if she couldn't breathe on her own soon, we might have to let her go. I decided, no more splitting my attention, no more conversations about 'what if'. I told my mum, "From this moment on, every ounce of my energy is going into Rambo." And I meant it.

For the next four days, I didn't leave the reception area. Same seat. Same spot. Twenty-four hours a day. Every four hours, she came out for a wee, tried to eat, and went back in. But something shifted. It was like she knew I was still there, through the night, through the fear, and she could finally rest enough to recover.

Slowly, her strength came back. She started taking food from my hand, breathing a little longer without oxygen, finding her spark again. And on the fourth day, she walked out of intensive care and came home with me, breathing on her own.

No one knows what caused the illness or why she turned a corner so suddenly. But I know this: sometimes the climb isn't about moving. It's about refusing to move away. It's about showing up in the same seat, over and over, until the fight comes back.

Rambo has been a picture of health and muscle ever since. And every time I see her chasing leaves, I'm reminded that your presence is sometimes the most powerful work you can do.

The Discipline That Carries You

There's a part of me that people don't always expect when they hear me talk about healing and growth. They see vulnerability, the tears, and the deep, reflective side of me. They don't always realise that this was built on a foundation of pain, precision and discipline.

I once climbed a mountain with thirty kilos on my back, a rifle strapped to me, in full military kit and with a broken leg. That wasn't inspiring. That was *necessary*. Giving up wasn't an option, not in the RAF. Not in my head. Not in the life I was living back then.

You never forget that kind of grit. You carry it. Sometimes it's not the journaling, or the reflection, or the emotional processing that gets you through. Sometimes, it's simply:

Shut up. Ruck up. Move forward.

No fanfare. No waiting for motivation. Just discipline.

David Goggins calls it the cookie jar – a mental vault where you keep the proof that you've survived worse. When your mind says you can't do it, you reach in and pull out a moment like that climb. That time you kept going anyway.

Jocko Willink says it even more simply: "Discipline equals freedom."

And he's right. Turns out, the stuff I least wanted to do was the stuff that set me free. Freedom doesn't come from comfort; it comes from choosing *hard things* on purpose. It comes from doing what your soul needs, even when your mind is screaming for ease.

That's the climb. It's not fluffy. It's not always emotional. Sometimes, it's just brutal repetition of the same hard thing, over and over, until it becomes who you are.

Choose Your Hard

> *"Life is one of two hard paths; there's only one that leads you to happiness."*

Here's something I've come to live by:

Not climbing is hard. So is climbing.
Living inauthentically is hard. So is stepping into your truth.
Staying broken is hard. So is healing.

You don't get to choose *whether* life is hard. You only get to choose which *kind* of hard is worth it. Pretending you're fine is the hardest lie to live with.

And for me? The pain of staying stuck in someone else's life was far worse than any mountain I've had to climb, broken leg or not.

Reflection: How to Keep Climbing

To close this chapter, I want to leave you with the first few steps to take right now.

You don't need a five-year plan – not now. You don't need to be fearless, certain or ready. You just need a reason and a rep. This climb is built on small, brutal, honest steps, and here are the five to take now. Use them. Write them. Live them.

1. **Define your North Star** – What is the life you want to build, not for others, but for you? Write it in present tense. Make it visceral. "I live with peace. I speak my truth. I walk into rooms as me, not a version."

2. **Train your discipline** – Motivation is a bonus. Discipline is a muscle. Set one non-negotiable action a day that pulls you forward and honour it like your life depends on it. Because maybe it does.
3. **Stack the proof** – Create a 'resilience resume'. List every moment you didn't think you could keep going but did. That's your ammo when fear starts talking.
4. **Reroute your inner voice** – When your mind says, "This is too hard," reply, "And I'm still doing it." When it says, "Who do you think you are?" answer, "Exactly who I say I am."
5. **Let the climb shape you** – Stop waiting for it to get easier. Start showing yourself how strong you've become.

And finally: **What version of me do I meet at the summit, and how do I start living like them now?**

This isn't a metaphor. This is your life. This is your climb.

When I think about this, I often think about those four days I refused to leave the vets while Rambo fought for her life. I wasn't climbing a literal mountain; I was sitting in the same chair, over and over. But I was still climbing.

Sometimes, the climb doesn't look like big leaps or grand gestures. Sometimes it's about staying when it's uncomfortable, exhausting, or when every part of you wants to run.

Your mountain might be a relationship, a business, a dream or your own recovery, but the principle is the same:

Be the one who doesn't walk away.

If you're still going, you're not behind. You're not broken. You're not lost.

You're climbing.

And that's the most courageous thing a person can do. Keep going. Do it scared. One foot in front of the other. The summit won't change you. The climb already is.

PART TWO

THE BECOMING

The becoming is where the real work begins. Not the leap, not the fall... the rebuilding. This part is quieter. But it's not gentle. It's confronting. It's heavy. It's honest. It's the part that asks you:

Who are you, really, when no one's watching?

What do you keep? What do you let go of? What do you *finally* stop apologising for?

No one sees it. There's no audience here. No standing ovation. No Instagram-worthy montage. Just you. Your truth. And the work.

The becoming doesn't happen in one lightning moment of clarity. It happens in a thousand small, unglamorous choices. It's you, choosing your future self, over and over again, even when the old one is clawing to stay alive.

This is the unbecoming of everything you thought you had to be, so you can become everything you were always meant to be. My parents often say to me now that they've seen the light come back in their child's eyes. Maybe that's what this whole thing is about, not becoming someone new, but letting the light back in.

This part can be electric.

Sure, it's hard, and you'll still have days you want to hide. But you'll also start to catch glimpses of yourself you've never seen before. A spark in your own eyes, a laugh that comes from somewhere deeper, a sudden moment where you realise: *I actually like who I'm becoming.*

These moments are gold. You'll want to bottle them. And the best part? They're only going to grow.

This is the Becoming.

If you've made it here, you've already proven you can do hard things. You've already leapt. You've already faced truths most people never touch. The rest? This is where we build the life that matches that kind of courage.

In the next chapters, we'll strip away what's been holding you back, step into the identity that belongs at the summit, and learn to live there, not just visit.

6

CHOOSING TO LEAP

WHEN 'NO MORE' BECOMES LOUDER THAN 'WHAT IF'

There's a moment – not always loud, not always dramatic – when the quiet becomes unbearable. You sit in your car a little too long after work. You catch your own eyes in the mirror and don't recognise them. You keep going through the motions of a life that, from the outside, might look fine… even successful. But something in you whispers, **"I can't do this anymore."**

Every turning point you've ever envied in someone else's story began with a whisper just like this. For you, it might be staring at a half-written resignation email you've opened every morning for six months. Or lying in bed at 2 am, rehearsing the breakup you still haven't had the guts to start. That moment isn't weakness. It's awareness. And awareness always comes before change.

But here's the truth: **Choosing to leap is terrifying.**

Because it means disappointing people, letting go of everything you worked for, and burning a life you built because it was slowly burning *you*. And it means being honest, for maybe the first time, about what you really want.

The Limit

When people say, "I hit rock bottom," what they mean is: *I ran out of energy to keep performing.*

The mask slipped. The story stopped working. The pain finally outran the excuses. For me, that limit looked like staring out over the edge of a life I could no longer survive in. Jess had run out of road. I wasn't making a choice between 'okay' and 'better'. I was choosing between a lie and a lifetime.

Your version might not look like mine. It could be the day you can't fake another smile at work, or when the thought of one more holiday with the in-laws makes your chest tighten.

Most people don't leap for a dream. They leap to survive.

Survival can look like smiling in family photos while secretly wishing you were somewhere else. It can look like answering emails with a tight chest. It can look like lying awake at night, rehearsing a life you don't even want.

You're not selfish for needing more. You're not ungrateful for wanting better. You're not broken because the life you built isn't enough anymore. You're just done with betraying yourself to keep everyone else comfortable.

The Fear of Disappointing Others

This one is brutal. Often, it's not the leap itself that scares us but the *reactions to it*. What will they think? What will they say? Will they still love me? Will I lose everyone?

It's not irrational; we are biologically wired to fear disconnection. As infants, disapproval could literally mean death. That wiring doesn't just disappear because we turn thirty. That's why a cold look from your boss or a sigh from your partner can feel like a punch in the gut. Your brain thinks your tribe might leave you behind.

So instead of leaping, we learn to perform. We become what people want us to be: the good one, the successful one, the strong one, the selfless one.

We don't ask, "Who am I?"

We ask, "Who do they need me to be?"

But here's what I've learned: **Disappointing others is a price worth paying if it means you stop disappointing yourself.**

If the cost of their comfort is your happiness, it's too expensive. And the people who love you for *who you really are?* They'll walk with you, even if they don't fully understand yet.

When Their Fear Becomes Yours

Sometimes the most paralysing fear doesn't even start with us. It starts with the people who love us projecting their fears onto our future.

> *"Are you sure?"*
> *"What if it doesn't work?"*
> *"Why can't you just be happy with what you've got?"*

They're not trying to hurt you. They're trying to keep you safe. But often, the safety they offer is just a mirror of their own limitations. It's like when someone tells you not to swim because they once saw a documentary about sharks. Their fear, not yours.

Here's what helped me:

I stopped trying to explain my freedom to people who had chosen their cages. I started letting love exist without needing understanding. You don't need to make everyone okay with your decision. (I know this is stupidly hard. I still struggle now, but it's true.) You just need to be okay with *why* you made it.

The Sunk Cost Fallacy

This is the lie that keeps people stuck for decades: **"I've already invested too much to walk away now."**

We say this about jobs, relationships, degrees, roles and identities, as if the time spent there justifies continuing the pain. But time invested is not the same as value created. You can pour your whole soul into something and still know it's not right. You can give years to a version of yourself and still outgrow it.

The bravest thing you can do is walk away *because* of how much you've given, not despite it, because you finally realise your investment doesn't demand your imprisonment. You are not abandoning what you've built. You are rescuing yourself from it.

You Don't Need a Guarantee

Here's what no one tells you before you leap. You won't feel ready. There is no 'right time'. No perfect sign. No sudden disappearance of fear.

There is only this: **You get to a point where not changing feels more dangerous than changing.**

And when it happens, you won't get fireworks. You'll just feel a quiet, stubborn clarity that you can't keep living like this. That's it. That's the moment.

Robin Sharma calls it, "the war between the voice of the soul and the voice of the ego."

The ego will beg you to stay comfortable. The soul will quietly remind you: this isn't where you belong. And most people wait. They wait for certainty and for courage. But you are never going to feel like it, so you must move anyway.

Make the Leap Personal

No one can leap for you. And no one should tell you where to leap to. This isn't about *their* mountain. This is about yours. You might leap into a new career, or out of a relationship. You might come out, like I did, and start your whole life again. You might leave a religion or a city, or just finally say, "I need help." If it's not your leap, it won't last.

Whatever it is, it has to be *your* truth, because when it gets hard, and it will, you need a reason strong enough to keep climbing. Jay Shetty says, "When you don't know what to do next, go back to your values." So start there. What matters more than comfort? More than applause? More than fitting in?

Let your leap come from the deepest part of you, the part that's still whispering, even after all this time.

Start Here

If you're standing on your own edge right now, here's what I want you to know:

>You are not too late.
>You are not too broken.
>You are not too much.
>You are **right on time.**

Fear doesn't mean you're on the wrong path; it means this path matters. And even if your legs are shaking, even if your hands are trembling, even if the fear is loud, you are allowed to choose yourself. You are allowed to want more. You are allowed to begin again.

And the sooner you do, the sooner the life you were meant to live can find you.

Reflection: What's My Leap?

Write these down. Sit with them. No pressure to answer perfectly. Just listen.

1. What area of my life feels most misaligned right now?
2. Am I holding on to something just because I've held it for so long?
3. Whose approval am I still trying to earn?
4. What would I choose if fear wasn't in the room?
5. Where am I ready to leap to… even if I'm scared?

7

THE FEAR SPECTRUM

HOW TO TELL THE DIFFERENCE BETWEEN PROTECTION AND PARALYSIS

The Fear That Keeps You Small vs The Fear That Moves You Forward

Your stomach drops. Your chest tightens. You can't tell if you're about to ruin your life… or save it. That's fear.

Fear has always had a seat at the table. It's just that for most of us, it's sitting at the head. The problem isn't fear; it's that we rarely stop to ask what *kind* of fear we're actually feeling. Is it the kind that's trying to save your life? Or the kind that's just trying to save your ego?

There's a difference. And learning that difference is one of the most powerful tools in your transformation. We're taught from a young age that all fear means 'stop'. That we shouldn't speak up. Don't stand out. Don't rock the boat. Don't chase the thing that might make people feel uncomfortable. Don't leave what's 'safe'.

But what if that kind of fear isn't a warning? What if it is a compass?

The Three Faces of Fear

Let's break fear down into three categories. I learned to identify these the hard way, and they still show up, even now.

1. Useful Fear

This is fear doing its job. It's the voice that stops you from walking down a dark alley at 3 am. The alert that makes you double-check the car door is locked. It's survival-driven and rooted in real danger.

Useful fear protects you. It's fast. It's instinctual. It's clear. If your gut says, "This isn't right," trust that. Your body is wired for threat detection, and when it's working from experience and evidence, it's wise.

As Gavin de Becker explains in *The Gift of Fear,* the more you learn to respect your intuition instead of ignoring it, the more you stay safe. Not by being paranoid, but by being attuned.

2. Irrational Fear

This one is trickier. It's fear that *feels* real but is based on stories, not facts.

It's the fear that says:

> "If I quit this job, I'll never succeed again."
> "If I leave this relationship, no one will ever love me."
> "If I come out, I'll lose everyone."

It's fear dressed as logic. But really? It's your nervous system clinging to the familiar. It sounds sensible. It's still a lie. This kind of fear isn't about protecting your life. It's about protecting your *identity*, even if that identity isn't truly you.

I faced this kind of fear when I stood in front of a mirror as Jess and admitted to myself that I was Jax. I knew my life would change. I knew it would be hard. But was the fear trying to save me?

No. It was trying to preserve the illusion, the old life. The 'fine' life. This kind of fear doesn't protect you from pain. It protects you from *growth*.

This is the same fear that stops you from raising your hand in a meeting because 'what if I sound stupid,' or keeps you from joining a gym because 'what if everyone looks at me'. None of those things is a life-or-death situation, but your brain treats them like they are.

3. Fear of Vulnerability

The third kind of fear? This is the most dangerous and the most powerful if you learn how to work with it.

This is the fear of being seen. Not the edited version. Not the curated story. You.

It's the fear that says:

> "If they see the real me, they'll leave."
> "If I show weakness, I lose power."

"If I tell the truth, I'll lose love."

It's the fear of walking into a room with no armour. Of letting your truth be heard without knowing how it will land. Of standing on stage, in your home, in your own skin and saying, *this is who I am.*

Sometimes, that fear shows up in ways that seem small from the outside, like the picture you've been waiting to post on social media. You've taken it, you love it, but you keep overthinking what people might say. You've rewritten the caption ten times. You've hovered over the 'share' button and backed out. It's not really about the photo. It's about the risk of being seen as you are, without the filters or the control. That hesitation is the same fear at work, the one that whispers, "What will they think?" every time you dare to show the unedited you. And the second you post it? That's you telling fear it doesn't get to drive.

This kind of fear doesn't mean you're weak. **It means you're getting closer to your power.**

No one explains this better than **Brené Brown.** In *The Call to Courage (Netflix)* she says:

"You can choose courage, or you can choose comfort. But you cannot choose both."

That stopped me cold. Because I'd lived my life trying to be both. I wanted to be brave but not too exposed. Real, but still liked. Authentic, but not rejected.

It doesn't work that way. Vulnerability isn't the opposite of strength; it *is* strength. It's the moment you show up without a guaranteed outcome. And that's what courage really is.

Vulnerability – *"Risk, uncertainty, and emotional exposure."*

Courage – *"Risk, uncertainty, and emotional exposure."*

That's what I felt when I told the truth for the first time. When I walked away from a life people clapped for but didn't see me in. When I let Jess go, and started becoming Jax, without knowing who'd stay.

And I'll tell you this with full honesty: the fear still shows up. But now, when it does? I listen. I breathe. And I walk forward *with it,* not away from it. Because that's what courage looks like.

The Fear of Being Seen

I've met some of the hardest men you can imagine. Men who've lived lives that would crush most people. But you know what's wild? Most of them are scared of the same thing we all are: being seen.

Let me tell you about a man we'll call John. I met him while working in the prison system. A grown man, built like a brick wall, bald head, tattoos, scars, history. He had experienced and witnessed things you couldn't begin to imagine. John had been in prison sixteen years at the point I met him, and he was one of the first prisoners I spoke to about what I was going through when I first returned to work and began to transition.

John came on that journey with me and, in the process, began to talk about his own trauma, took accountability and did the inner work that was necessary for him to stop taking drugs, self-harming and resorting to violence as a coping mechanism. About twelve months into my transition, I held a transgender awareness event at the prison to thank them for supporting me throughout this process.

The event had around one hundred and fifty members of staff present, and the only prisoners allowed to attend were the residents of the PIPE Unit *(Psychologically Informed Planned Environment)* that I worked on. I had T-shirts made for them to wear, specifically as they had also been on this journey with me. The T-shirts all had a butterfly on the front, and each had a saying that I live by on the back. One shirt said: Feel the fear and do it anyway. The second shirt said: Remember who you are. And the third said: Be unapologetically you.

John came up to me on the morning of the event and said, "Mr Feeley, I'm going to wear a jumper underneath my T-shirt."

Bear in mind, this was the height of summer. I asked John why he wanted to do that, to which he replied, "Well, I've never left the wing in sixteen years without long sleeves on," because of the serious self-harm scars on his arms.

Me: What does that T-shirt say on the back?

John: Be unapologetically you.

Me: Right then, what do we always talk about? Those scars are part of you and your story. They represent everything that tried to beat you. You go up there and you show everyone how much you have completely changed your life around. Never be ashamed of your past or anything about who you are: it got you to where you are right now."

John stood up in front of one hundred and fifty prison officers that day and told them he wasn't ashamed of his scars anymore because they were part of his story. In his words, "Mr Feeley saved my life."

This story doesn't sound like much. But it was massive. For both John and me. He showed up differently from that day. Not fixed, but seen.

We think vulnerability is weakness. We think it's 'soft'. But I'm telling you now, that moment between me and John was one of the most courageous things I've ever witnessed.

And here's the lesson:

You showing up as the real you might be the permission someone else needs to do the same. That's why we have to challenge the fear of being vulnerable. Sometimes, your scars become someone else's survival guide.

That's not poetry. That's survival.

I've always worn my heart on my sleeve, literally. When I was in my early twenties, I scribbled a rough sketch of a love heart on a piece of paper and had it tattooed on my arm. It's not polished or perfect, but it's mine.

For me, it's a reminder to lead with love, always. To stay open, even when it would be easier to close myself off. Every time I look at it, I'm reminded that I would rather risk getting hurt than live guarded and untouched. That doesn't mean I haven't been hurt; I have, deeply. But shutting down would mean losing the best parts of myself.

It's like having animals. I have two dogs that I love deeply, an eight-year-old Hungarian Vizsla named Rocky and a five-year-old Weimaraner named Rambo. They're basically my children, and pretty much the dog versions of me: big ears, long arms and daft as a brush. We open ourselves up to loving pets, knowing damn well they're going to break our hearts one day. But the happiness, joy and unconditional love they bring to our lives are worth all the heartache in the world.

Wearing your heart on your sleeve, whether it's scars or tattoos, is a form of vulnerability. It tells the world: *This is who I am. I'm not hiding it to make you comfortable.* And that's terrifying, because love, in any form, means there are no guarantees. You can't armour up and fully connect at the same time.

But the times I've shown my heart, despite the terror? Those are the moments that have led to the most connection, the most growth, and the most happiness, both in me and in the people who saw it and thought, *maybe I can do that too.*

That's the thing about vulnerability: it's never just about you. Your willingness to be seen gives others permission to be seen. And the moment you start leading with what's real, flaws and all, is the moment fear stops being the enemy… and starts becoming the indicator that you're exactly where you need to be.

Fear Isn't the Enemy. It's the Indicator.

The most dangerous thing about fear isn't how it feels. It's how it quietly runs your life when you don't know it's driving.

Most people aren't choosing the wrong life out of spite or stupidity. They're choosing it because they've mistaken *safety* for *peace.* They've confused *discomfort* with *danger.*

But fear isn't a stop sign. It's a signal. A signpost pointing towards the edge of your comfort zone and the beginning of freedom.

Here's what I know now:

    Useful fear keeps you alive.
    Irrational fear keeps you stuck.

Vulnerable fear? That's the one that will set you free… if you let it.

You'll never be fearless. You're not supposed to be.

But if you can learn to ask if this fear is protecting you, or just protecting the version of you that you've outgrown, you'll start making decisions based on *truth*, not trauma.

Reflection: Which Fear Are You Feeding?

To finish this chapter, take a few moments to check in with yourself.

Write down or sit with these questions:

1. What fear am I facing right now?
2. Which category does it belong in? Is it useful, irrational or vulnerable?
3. What has this fear cost me so far?
4. What would it feel like to do the thing anyway?
5. Who else might find courage if I go first?

You're not weak for feeling fear. You're human. But you are powerful when you stop letting it be the loudest voice in the room. And maybe… you're not scared of falling. Maybe you're scared of flying.

Fear is not the enemy. It's just the guard dog. Train it to walk beside you… and it will follow you through any door you choose to open.

8

LIVING BY DESIGN, NOT DEFAULT

CHOOSING WHAT'S YOURS TO CARRY

There's a moment on the journey – after the chaos, after the grief, after the fear – when you stop running from your old life… and start sorting through it. Not everything has to go. Not everything deserves to stay. The power is in choosing. Because here's the truth: **most people don't create their life. They inherit it.**

They inherit their beliefs. Their values. Their roles. Their limits. Their labels. They don't build a life, they *maintain* one. An inherited life can feel deceptively safe because it comes pre-approved. But approval isn't the same as alignment, and safety isn't the same as freedom. And since you're here, I'm guessing that's not enough for you anymore.

Earlier, in Chapter Three, we discussed **The Sorting Table.** Imagine walking into a room filled with everything that's made you who you are. Memories. Beliefs. Habits. People. Labels. Roles. Stories. All laid out in front of you like evidence from your life.

Now imagine browsing those tables with two boxes in hand:

One box is labelled **'Keep'**. The other is labelled **'Let Go.**

For the first time, *you* get to decide what goes where.

This isn't about burning your past to the ground. It's about honouring it, learning from it, and *releasing* what no longer fits. Think of it like renovating a house. You don't bulldoze the whole thing just because some walls are cracked. You strip out the mould, open the windows and rebuild the parts that can actually hold you.

What You Keep

You keep what's real. This means the things that feel like *home*, not like performance. The values that still hold weight. The people who love the unmasked version of you. The tools that serve your future, not just your survival.

You keep the resilience you earned, the compassion you fought for, and the lessons pain taught you. You also keep the proof, the reminders, of every time you thought you couldn't, but did. Those memories become anchors in your next storm.

Just because something came from a hard place doesn't mean it's worthless. Some of your strongest traits were born in fire. You don't have to throw them out, just learn to *carry them differently.*

What You Lose

You lose what was never really yours. This includes the pressure to always be 'fine', the guilt that kept you small, the job title that became your identity, the need to be liked more than understood, and the friendships that only exist because you kept pretending.

You also let go of survival mechanisms dressed up as personality traits. This is the tricky part, because letting go of these can feel like letting go of yourself. But you're not erasing who you are. You're releasing the costumes you wore to get through. You release the people-pleasing, the over-functioning and the perfectionism.

I once heard Matthew Hussey say, "You're not a bad person for who you had to become to survive. But you're allowed to outgrow that version of you."

You're Not Starting From Scratch

This is important: you're not starting over. **You're starting fresh – with experience.**

Think of your growth like building muscle. You don't throw your old body away. You adapt it. You stress it in the right places. You rest. You rebuild.

Same goes here.

You're not erasing who you were. You're evolving it. The pain, the wins, the heartbreak, the healing, they all come with you. Not to weigh you down… but to remind you how far you've already come.

The Myth of Overnight Change

Let's kill a myth while we're here: You don't have to reinvent your life in one dramatic, cinematic moment. Change doesn't always feel like a breakthrough. Sometimes it feels like boredom. Like repetition. Like choosing the better option on a Wednesday when nobody's watching.

As James Clear says in *Atomic Habits*, "Every action you take is a vote for the type of person you wish to become."

Not a grand gesture. A vote. And sometimes, that single vote, that single choice, matters far more than you think.

It reminds me of a story Barack Obama tells us about a woman named Edith Child, a retired librarian who knocked on doors every day during one of Obama's campaigns. She showed up no matter what: rain, snow or blistering heat. One afternoon, a young man finally answered his door after weeks of ignoring her. She asked him if he was going to vote, and he shrugged. She told him that one voice can change a conversation, one conversation can change a mind, and one mind can change a community.

This man showed up on election day. And when the votes were counted, the margin in that district was a single vote.

We think change is made by sweeping movements or big breaks. But more often, it's made by the small, steady voices that refuse to go away. One vote rarely changes an election, but hundreds of votes do. That's how you become someone new: not with one leap, but with enough tiny votes cast for the person you're becoming.

Change happens in tiny, almost invisible decisions. It is in choosing the hard conversation. In walking away when it would be easier to stay. In showing up as the real you, even when it's awkward. In saying 'no' without explanation. That's the work. Not the highlight reel, but the hidden habits.

In the words of Barack Obama himself, "One voice can change a room. And if it can change a room, it can change a city. And if it can change a city, it can change a state. If it can change a state, it can change a nation. And if it can change a nation, it can change the world."

Humour Helps

Let's be real: this stuff gets heavy. Some days you'll feel like a monk. Other days you'll feel like a walking contradiction. You're human. Laugh at it. Laugh at *yourself*.

One of the best signs that you're healing is when you can look back and smile. Not because it was funny, but because you're no longer stuck in it.

> *"The person who falls and gets up is much stronger than the person who never fell."*
>
> **– Robin Sharma**

And the person who can laugh at the fall? That's next level.

What Will You Carry?

Here's your chance to start sorting through everything in that room. Not to impress anyone. Not to prove your worth. Just to get *honest*.

Ask yourself:

1. What parts of me feel heavy? What parts feel like home?
2. Which values do I live by and which ones were I just handed?
3. Who makes me feel more like myself? Who makes me shrink?
4. What habits are building the future I want? Which ones are numbing me from it?
5. If I could rebuild my life like a house, what would I lay as a foundation?

There are no perfect answers. The power lies in the act of *asking*.

Reflection: Your Keep and Let Go Lists

Try this:

Draw a line down the middle of a page. Label one side 'Keep' and the other 'Let Go'. Then list *everything*: traits, beliefs, relationships, roles, habits… and sort honestly.

Come back to your lists often. It's not a one-time thing. It's a lifelong practice. A recalibration.

Becoming isn't a destination. It's a commitment to never again carrying what isn't truly yours.

9

BEYOND THE QUIET

WHERE STILLNESS TURNS INTO STRENGTH

The quiet can break you before it builds you. And no one warns you about it.

If the leap is the spark, the hard middle is the forge. It's where the heat is steady, not spectacular. It's where you're not celebrated for jumping anymore, you're tested for staying.

The first time you find yourself in the quiet, it feels like a cliff drop. You're standing there without all the noise, the job, the relationships, the constant proving, and the silence feels almost unbearable.

But the second time? The second time is different. The second time, you step into the quiet on purpose. And that's when the *real* work begins. Because in Part One, sitting in the quiet was about survival. It was about learning to be *with* yourself at all. Here in Part Two, the quiet isn't accidental. It's intentional. It's where you *build*.

This is the chapter no one glamorises. Because this part is where you face the parts of yourself that don't dissolve just because you made a leap. This is where you start laying brick on brick to create the version of you that can hold the life you've been fighting for.

Why It Feels Harder Before It Gets Easier

We think that once we've made the leap, the hard part is over. That once we've stripped away the noise and found the courage to sit still, the rest will be peaceful. But I want to tell you the truth:

The quiet will often feel harder before it feels better.

Why? Because your nervous system is adjusting to a new normal. The noise, even the painful, stressful, chaotic noise, used to give you something to hold on to. A role. A distraction. An identity.

Now, without the constant rush, without the external distractions, you're face to face with the deeper work, and that work doesn't scream, it whispers. It whispers all the truths you've ignored. The fears you buried. The old wounds that never got closure.

This is why so many people run back to old habits during this stage. Not because they want the old life back, but because the quiet makes them feel raw, exposed and uncertain.

The Pull Back to Chaos

Why does your brain try to drag you back to the life you outgrew?

The pull back to chaos is sneaky, and it often disguises itself as nostalgia, logic or even 'self-awareness'.

After you leap, after you make the choice, after you leave the job, the relationship, the identity, there will be a moment, maybe days or even months later, when you feel an almost magnetic pull back to what you left.

It won't make sense logically. You *know* it wasn't right. You *know* it was suffocating you. But the thought comes in anyway: *"Was it really that bad? Maybe I overreacted. Maybe I could make it work."*

This is the first thing I want you to know:

The urge is not proof that you made the wrong choice. It's proof that your nervous system is recalibrating. Think of it like quitting sugar; the cravings peak just as your body starts healing. Your brain isn't asking for the old life because it was better. It's asking because it doesn't yet know how to feel safe without it.

Why Familiar Chaos Feels Safer Than Peace

Our brains are wired for familiarity, not happiness. It's a survival mechanism. Your nervous system learned a long time ago how to operate in chaos, in tension, in discomfort. It knows the rules there. Even if that chaos was toxic, it was predictable. And the human brain *loves* predictability, because predictability feels safe.

This is why people leave relationships that hurt them, only to end up back with the same person. It is why people quit jobs they hated, only to return to the same industry that burned them out. It is also why people walk away from an old version of themselves, only to start performing again for someone new.

It's not weakness. It's wiring.

Attachment and the Myth of 'Going Back'

Attachment theory explains so much of this. If you grew up learning that love, safety, or approval was inconsistent, if you had to work for it, fight for it, or shape-shift to keep it… discomfort became your normal. So, when life gets quiet, when it gets steady, when there's *no* chaos to manage, your system panics. It mistakes the absence of drama for the absence of safety.

You end up rewriting the story of your past, editing out the parts that hurt, romanticising the parts that felt like connection, convincing yourself the old life was better than it was. I've been there so many times, whether it was a relationship, a career choice or my identity. Late at night, I scrolled through old photos, wondering if I'd made a huge mistake. Familiar pain felt safer than foreign peace.

So many people finally leave that corporate job they hate so much, the one that drained them of every ounce of energy, to end up back on LinkedIn six weeks later, tempted to apply for the same type of role. Not because they miss the work, but because they miss the certainty of knowing exactly who they had to be every day.

Nostalgia Isn't Truth, It's a Filter

The problem is, when we feel lost in the hard middle, the brain edits our memories. Psychologists call this *nostalgia bias*.

You remember the highs, but you often soften the lows. You tell yourself, "Maybe it wasn't so bad."

But here's the truth:

If it was enough to make you leap, it was enough to keep you moving forward. That old life didn't suddenly become the right fit just because the new life feels uncomfortable. The discomfort you're in now is growth. The discomfort you were in before was survival.

Would you really be happy if you went back? How did you feel when you were there? Is that what you really want? Or is this bit just really hard?

The Hardest Truth

Sometimes peace feels boring. Sometimes stability feels hollow. Sometimes growth feels lonelier than the chaos ever did.

That doesn't mean you're on the wrong path. It means you're building tolerance for a life you've never lived before. Your nervous system is learning that peace isn't danger, that stillness isn't punishment, and that love or self-worth doesn't need to be earned through pain.

Your Anchor When You Want to Go Back

Whenever you feel that pull to go back, ask yourself:

> *Am I missing the person, or the pattern?*
> *Am I longing for the old life, or the feeling of certainty I had there?*
> *If I went back, would I be going back to comfort or to truth?*

Write these down. Keep them close. The urge to return will come in waves, especially in the quiet. And every time it does, remember that going back won't give you peace. It will just delay the climb you know you're here to make.

If you need something tangible in those moments, try one of these:

- Keep a photo or note in your phone titled 'Why I Left'. Read it when you're tempted to go back.
- Call or message a 'future you' friend, someone who reminds you where you're heading.
- Change your environment for ten minutes. Walk, shower or drive to break the nostalgia loop in your brain.
- Play a song that represents freedom to you; it can reset your emotional state faster than you think.

When the pull feels strongest, you're not weak; you're on the verge of rewiring. Every time you choose to stay, you're teaching your nervous system: 'This is safe now'. That's how the old world loses its grip.

When I think about songs that anchor me, I always go back to one moment when I was about fourteen. I was a young girl in high school, already fighting the kind of battles that don't always leave visible bruises, the daily grind of mental bullying, the quiet cruelty teenagers can be so skilled at. I was just trying to find my place in the world. I'd always been physically tough, but I was shy and sensitive. One day, my dad played me a song I'd never heard before: *The Gambler* by Kenny Rogers.

It wasn't a love song. Nor was it a motivational anthem in the usual sense. It was a conversation between two strangers on a train, one passing down his life philosophy to the other. The chorus still plays in my head:

> *"You've got to know when to hold 'em, know when to fold 'em, know when to walk away, and know when to run."*

At fourteen, I didn't know much about poker (I still don't), but I knew what it felt like to want to fight every battle, answer every insult, prove myself to people determined not to see me. I also knew how it felt to stay in the shadows, keep quiet and let people walk all over me. My dad told me, "Life isn't about reacting to everything that's thrown at you. It's about knowing which hands are worth playing."

That song taught me something I still carry, especially now in the online world, when people's opinions fly at you like cards across the table. You can't play every hand. You can't meet every challenge with a fight. Sometimes, strength is holding your ground. Sometimes it's walking away before you lose more than the game. And sometimes, it's running with your peace intact.

The Psychology of the Hard Middle

Why it feels like you're going backwards:

The middle isn't just about pushing forward. It's about *fighting the pull backwards*. And that pull? It's strong. Sometimes stronger than the push forward.

It's a bit like stretching out a rubber band behind you as you move. Every step forward creates tension, and that tension makes you feel like, at any moment, you'll be snapped right back to where you started. That's why the middle feels so exhausting. You're not only moving towards the new, you're resisting the magnetic pull of the old.

And here's the truth that most people don't say out loud: sometimes just staying where you are, without snapping back, is progress. Standing still can be just as much of an achievement as making leaps forward. If all you did today was stop yourself from falling back into old patterns, that's not weakness — that's strength.

My Experience in the Deep Work

I remember a few months into my transition, I thought I'd already done the hardest bit. I'd leapt. I'd faced the world as Jax. I'd sat through the grief of losing my identity as Jess. And yet, this was the period that nearly broke me. I had no idea that the work I needed to do had only just begun. And it was slowly getting worse before it was to get better.

The initial adrenaline of survival had worn off. There were no big 'milestone' wins every week to keep me fuelled. There was just… me and the daily repetitive work of rebuilding my life in this new version of me as a person I didn't even know yet.

This is when I realised that big change doesn't happen when you jump. Big change happens in the consistency of the deep work when no one is watching. It's when you're tired. When you're bored. When no one's clapping. When no one's asking how you are anymore.

That's when the new life is built, not in the fire, but in the slow burn. How long it takes, we never know; we must just trust the process.

Why Support Matters Here

I want to be clear that this stage is vulnerable.

In my talks, I've often said that this middle ground is one of the most dangerous places for people, because you're stripped of your old coping mechanisms, but your new identity isn't fully formed yet. You're in no man's land.

And in that space, the temptation to go back to the relationship, to the job, to the old habits can feel overwhelming. You will do anything to shut that voice up in your mind.

That's why I'll say this: Please get help.

It doesn't make you weak. It keeps you safe. This might mean therapy, coaching, support groups, a mentor, or even one friend you can text to say, *"Today feels heavy."*

You are not meant to hold this stage alone. Even the most self-reliant people need a witness in this stage, someone to remind them of the road they've already walked when their own memory turns against them.

How to Endure the Hard Middle

This stage will test you in ways the leap never could. The leap is fuelled by adrenaline. This middle stage? It's fuelled by discipline.

You don't wake up with big cinematic breakthroughs. You wake up to the same feelings, the same fears, the same uncertainty, and the only thing that moves you forward is choosing the work again and again.

This is where most people quit, not because they aren't capable, but because they expected progress to *feel* better. They thought they'd have proof by now that the climb was worth it. But the proof comes *after* the consistency, not before. Motivation is unreliable here. It will disappear the second things get uncomfortable. Discipline is what carries you.

One of the best lessons I ever learned, from the RAF, from the Prison Service, from life, is that discipline beats motivation every time.

I've carried those words with me in more ways than one. In fact, they're inked permanently on my arms, a quote from the famous *Rocky* film: *"The world ain't all sunshine and rainbows; it's a very mean and nasty place, and I don't care how tough you are, it will beat you to your knees and keep you there if you let it. You, me or nobody is gonna hit as hard as life. But it ain't about how hard you hit, it's about how hard you can get hit and keep moving forward, how much you can take and keep moving forward. That is how winning is done."*

I was barely twenty when I had it done, but even back then, those words were armour. It was like a code between me and my dad. Every time I was going through something tough, physically, mentally or emotionally, he'd say those words to me.

In military training, on days when I thought I couldn't take another step, I'd hear that voice reminding me: life is all about how you keep moving forward. Even now, when my mind gets loud or the climb feels impossible, it's still there as my reminder that the fight isn't in the punches you throw, it's in the days you refuse to quit.

This is the mindset the Hard Middle demands. Not punishment. Not toxic grind. Just the quiet, repeated decision: *I'm doing the next step.* It is never about feeling ready. It's about doing the thing anyway - scared, tired and uncertain.

The Traps of the Hard Middle

Your brain is going to play tricks on you.

> *"It shouldn't be this hard by now."*
> *"If I was on the right path, it would feel easier."*
> *"Maybe this isn't working at all."*

I promise you this is normal. I still experience this now, wondering if I'm getting anywhere, if I'm helping anybody, having any impact at all. I ask myself constantly whether I should think of a new career path and focus on that. But I must constantly remind myself and sometimes those around me that I am in the messy middle. I am doubting myself in a lonely period of quiet and a million questions. And as uncomfortable as it is, that is okay, as long as I don't give up.

This is a psychological dip most people face when the novelty of change wears off and the work becomes repetitive. James Clear calls it *The Valley of Disappointment,* where the results aren't visible yet, but the effort is heavy. This is where people go back. Not because their old life was better, but because it was familiar.

What Success Looks Like Here

Most people misunderstand what success in the hard middle looks like. It doesn't look like fireworks. It doesn't look like applause. It looks like:

>Turning up to therapy when you'd rather cancel.
>Going to the gym even if you leave after ten minutes.
>Saying 'no' to the old patterns one more time.
>Choosing the new life *quietly* every day.

You might not feel like you're transforming. But one day, you'll look back and realise that every small, unglamorous choice was laying the foundations for the person you've become.

Becoming

This stage is uncomfortable because it's *rewriting you* at a core level.

At the start of change, you're still running on the old self's fuel, old habits, old adrenaline, old patterns that powered you to jump in the first place. But now? Those have burned out. You're left with the raw, exposed version of yourself that isn't fully built yet. It feels awkward. It feels unstable. And that's exactly what transformation feels like.

You are literally becoming someone new, but paradoxically that someone was in you all along. The hard middle isn't about inventing yourself from scratch. This stage is less like building a house from the ground up, and more like stripping wallpaper from an old room, layer by stubborn layer, until you finally see the wall you always knew was there. It's about removing everything that isn't really you, layer by layer, choice by choice.

Why It Feels Heavy

Psychologically, your brain is resisting because it doesn't fully trust this new identity yet.

> It wants to test you: "Are we really doing this?"
> It wants to keep you safe: "We could go back. That was easier."
> It wants certainty: "Prove to me this will work before I commit."

But identity doesn't work like that. Your mind doesn't shift by evidence first. Your mind shifts by *action first, evidence later.*

This is why the middle feels exhausting: you're showing up without proof yet. You're building self-trust without constant validation.

Living Like the Person You're Becoming

This stage is about congruence, living as the person you want to become *before* the world catches up.

Ask yourself:

> How would the version of me at the summit make decisions today?
> How would they treat themselves on hard days?
> What boundaries would they set?

And then, act accordingly.

At first, it feels forced. Like trying on clothes that don't quite fit yet. But every time you choose alignment, you're breaking in that identity until one day it's not 'becoming' anymore, it's just *you*.

When It Starts to Lift

Here's the funny thing about this stage: you won't notice the shift when it happens. It's not fireworks. It's not a lightning bolt. It's quiet. One day, you catch yourself laughing, not because you tried to, but because it just happened. One day, you walk past an old trigger, and it doesn't rip you apart like it used to.

That's how change arrives in the hard middle, not as a wave, but as ripples. Tiny, almost unnoticeable moments when the weight lightens. And you don't notice yourself rising... until you realise, you're no longer drowning.

So many people used to say to me in that first twelve months of transitioning: *"It's crazy how you can't see the weight on someone's shoulders until it's gone."* They never would've known I was drowning, until it became so obvious that I wasn't anymore.

Why This Stage Matters Most

This stage, more than the leap, more than the early quiet, more than the adrenaline of big change… this is where your real strength is forged. Here, in the middle, you are building the kind of resilience that doesn't come from one act of bravery but from a thousand quiet acts of self-respect.

> When you show up for yourself *without proof…*
> When you keep going *without applause…*
> When you choose alignment *without certainty…*

That's when you become unshakable. The middle is not the punishment. The middle is the making of you.

A Subtle Shift in Identity

You don't notice it straight away, but something else is happening in this stage. Your old self stops trying to pull you back quite so hard.

It's not that the nostalgia disappears; it's that you've started building a life that feels safer than the past. Your nervous system starts to catch up. Your mind starts to trust the new normal. And with that, your identity begins to shift. You're no longer someone who *is trying* to change. You are someone who *is changed*. When that realisation hits you, even in the smallest way, it's like reaching the first ledge on the climb back up.

I sometimes think back to that car journey with my mum, the one I told you about in Chapter Five, when *The Climb* came on the radio. Neither of us spoke; we just sat there, tears in our eyes, feeling the weight of what was ahead. Back then, I thought it was about that one mountain. That one leap. That one moment.

Now I know it was about all of them. The climbs I could see and the ones that came out of nowhere. The ones I chose and the ones that chose me. Every single one has shaped me. Every single one has been worth it.

And if I've learned anything, it's that there will always be another climb. The point isn't to get to the top and be done. The point is to keep showing up, one foot in front of the other, ready for whatever summit is next.

Reflection: A Check-In for the Hard Middle

If you're in the messy middle right now, I want you to pause and ask yourself the following questions:

1. What one small sign do you have that things are shifting? (It doesn't need to be huge. Sometimes it's just, "I don't react the way I used to.")
2. What is one habit that's keeping you anchored? (No overhauls, just one action that gives you a sense of stability.)
3. Who or what can I lean on this week when it feels heavy?
4. What proof can I stack from my past that I've done hard things before?

The middle is hard. That's why most people don't make it through. But if you are here, still moving, still showing up, you are already doing the thing most people won't.

You are not failing. You are becoming.

And the climb back up? It's already started.

You don't have to see the summit yet. You only have to know you're higher than you were yesterday. Because one day, without warning, you'll look up and realise you've been standing on solid ground for a while now.

10

THE CLIMB BACK UP

OWNING EVERY STEP YOU'VE FOUGHT FOR

The Reality of the Summit

Here's the truth about the top of the mountain: it's a liar. You think it's one final peak, but it's just another ledge before the next climb.

You'll think, "This is it, I've made it." And then life will hand you another incline. That's not failure. That's life.

Because the summit you're reaching for isn't a single point on a mountain. It's every step you take from which you can look back at where you were, and think: *I can't believe I made it here.*

When you've been through the quiet, the grief, the fear, and the messy middle, every ledge feels like a summit. And each one matters.

Looking Back

There's a psychological reason this is so important.

Humans are wired with negativity bias; we remember pain more vividly than progress. It's why, even halfway up the mountain, we convince ourselves we've made no progress at all. That's why you have to stop and look back. You will walk past versions of yourself you once prayed to become and not even notice. In the climb, you've **got to notice.**

Look back at the you who was just trying to survive. The you who couldn't sit still for five minutes. The you who thought they'd never take the leap, let alone survive it. They would look at you now, battered, tired, still moving and think: *You're incredible.*

That matters. Every day you keep moving forward is a day you make the younger you proud.

The Future Summits

The climb back up tricks you. The horizon plays games. You hit a ledge and your heart leaps; this must be the top. Then you crest it, and there it is: another stretch, another incline. Not failure. Just the truth about real growth.

Here's the paradox of the climb: you don't even know some of the summits that are waiting for you.

If someone had told me five years ago that I'd be speaking on stages and changing lives, or that my making all those scary decisions and steps in my life would help prisoners and people online save their own lives too, I would have laughed them out of the room.

Back then, my summit was just: *Make it through this alive.*

Every summit you reach shows you another peak you couldn't see from the bottom.

And here's what's even crazier: the higher you climb, the more it stops being about one final destination. It becomes about the process itself. The person you're becoming. The view from *each* point and enjoying the journey every step of the way.

The Psychology of Moving Forward

When we stop having a clear summit, we often fall into the arrival fallacy. The arrival fallacy is the belief that when we get there, we'll finally be happy.

But neuroscience is clear: when you hit a goal, your brain's reward system gives you a dopamine spike... and then resets. That's why even big wins can feel strangely anticlimactic. That's why the climb isn't just about the summit, it's about building a life that feels like you're summiting all the time. It's about learning to love the climb itself.

True happiness is in your daily life, not in a single moment. That's discipline. That's resilience. That's a sustainable life.

Living at the Summit
(without losing the climb)

The danger of the summit is comfort. And comfort can quietly turn into stagnation. That's why you keep finding new summits. Not because you're ungrateful. Not because you're broken. But because growth is the most natural human state there is.

I remember hearing Jay Shetty say, "The day you stop climbing is the day you start dying." I've lived that. That doesn't mean you never rest. It means you rest with intention. You pause, you breathe, you take in the view, then you set your sights on the next peak.

You are not at the mercy of the mountain; the mountain is at the mercy of you.

Reflection: Your Next Summit

I want you to write this down. Take a page and answer honestly:

1. What is my current summit? (What am I working towards now, not because I 'should', but because it calls me?)
2. What summits have I already reached that I haven't celebrated? (Make yourself name them.)
3. What values will guide my next climb?
4. What is one step I can take this week towards the next peak?

A Personal Note

If you take one thing from this book, let it be this:

You don't need to be fearless to climb. You just need to keep moving.

Fear, fatigue, uncertainty… they all come with you. But so does resilience. So does everything you've built in the quiet.

The climb back up is not about proving to the world that you can do it. It's about proving to *yourself* that you already are.

And the summit? It won't change you. The climb already has.

One Last Thing Before You Go

If you've made it here, to the final page, please take a second and realise something. You didn't just read this book. You walked through fire with me. You stood on the edge. You sat in the silence. You clawed your way through the climb. You did the heavy sorting, the grieving, the truth-telling.

And now… here you are. Still breathing. Still becoming. Still going.

You've already done the hardest part: you *stayed* with yourself. When most people run, distract, deny, or give up, *you stayed*. And that matters more than you think.

This book was never just about *my* leap. It's about *yours*.

I didn't write this to be inspirational. I wrote it to be a mirror, to reflect back to you the power that's already in you. The fire that's always been burning underneath all the noise.

You might not have all the answers yet. You might still be in the middle. You might still feel scared as hell. But that doesn't mean you're not ready. It means you're *real*. And real is always ready enough.

Let the world catch up later. Let the doubt shout if it wants. But from this moment forward, you walk into every room, not with certainty, not with perfection, but with truth. With your chest out, your voice steady (or shaking, that's okay too), and your soul completely unhidden.

You don't need permission anymore.

This is your permission.

>To keep growing.
>To keep healing.
>To keep becoming.

The world doesn't need more perfect people. It needs more honest ones. And you, my friend, are the real deal. Go live like it.

When you start to doubt yourself, when your legs shake, when your lungs burn, and when the summit feels too far away, remember this:

You've already survived everything that tried to break you. This mountain doesn't stand a chance.

You've already walked through fire. You've already stood on cliffs you thought would swallow you whole. And you're still here.

The mountain doesn't get the final say; you do. Not because you're fearless. Not because you're certain. But because you've decided to keep moving.

Do it shaking. Do it tired.

DO IT SCARED.

This mountain was never here to stop you. It was here to show you who you really are.

ABOUT THE AUTHOR

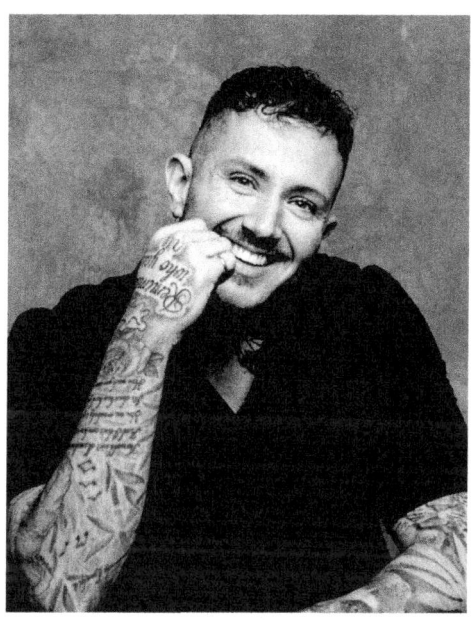

Jaxon Feeley has lived through the kind of fear most people hope they'll never face. He has served in the Royal Air Force, stood on prison landings with some of the UK's most dangerous individuals, and navigated a public gender transition under the spotlight of national media. Featured on Channel 4's BAFTA-nominated *Banged Up*, crowned a winner of *Hunted*, and heard on shows such as Virgin Radio and the *Homosapiens* podcast, Jax has become a recognised voice on courage, authenticity, and living your truth.

But *Fear Proof* is not a story about him - it's about you. In these pages, Jax shows that you don't need to be fearless to change your life; you just need the courage to ***do it scared.*** Drawing on raw experience, honest lessons, and a refusal to let fear dictate his future, he offers readers a blueprint for letting go, beginning again, and finally building a life that feels like home.

For more information or to contact Jax:

- 🌐 www.jaxonfeeley.com
- 📷 @jaxryderfeeley [Instagram]
- ♪ @jaxryderfeeley [TikTok]
- 📘 @Jaxon Feeley [Facebook]
- 💼 @Jaxon Feeley [LinkedIn]
- ▶ @Jaxon Feeley [YouTube]

Printed in Dunstable, United Kingdom